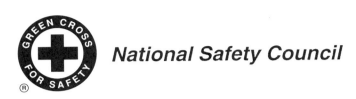 **National Safety Council**

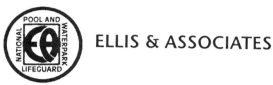 **ELLIS & ASSOCIATES**

INSTRUCTOR'S RESOURCE MANUAL
FOR THE
LEARN TO SWIM
PROGRAM

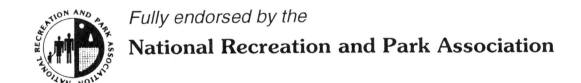 *Fully endorsed by the*
National Recreation and Park Association

Editorial, Sales, and Customer Service Offices
Jones and Bartlett Publishers
40 Tall Pine Drive
Sudbury, MA 01776
(508) 443-5000
(800) 832-0034

Jones and Bartlett Publishers International
Barb House, Barb Mews
London W6 7PA
UK

ISBN 0-7637-0221-8

The information presented in this book is based on the most recent recommendations of responsible medical/industrial sources. The National Safety Council, the authors and the publisher, however, make no guarantee as to, and assume no responsibility for, correctness, sufficiency, or completeness of such information or recommendations. Other or additional measures may be required under particular circumstances. The CPR material is provided by Jeff Ellis & Associates, International Consultant for Aquatic Safety.

Printed in the United States of America
00 99 98 97 96   10 9 8 7 6 5 4 3 2 1

Contents

PART FOUR - ADAPTED AQUATICS PROGRAM

Foreword

You are about to depart on a new professional Journey - that of becoming a National Safety Council Learn to Swim Instructor. If this is your first time at teaching aquatic skills, or if you are an experienced aquatic professional, we hope that the Learn to Swim Instructor training program will broaden your horizons and expand your perspective.

As you become familiar with the components of the Learn to Swim program, you will begin to understand the philosophy and foundation that makes this program so special and full of potential for your facility and the patrons you serve. Some of the unique features include:
- flexibility
- measurable Standards of Care
- system of accountability
- focus on the learner, not the teacher
- developmentally appropriate
- breaking down learning barriers for accelerated progress
- integrated programs offering the full spectrum of aquatic instruction-Exploration, Journey, Challenge and Adapted

You will also be able to tailor your instructor training requirements to meet a level appropriate to the student's age, physical, and emotional levels. For example, you do not have to be trained in the entire Learn to Swim program if your talent and objectives are to teach only ages 4-7 in the Journey One level. This flexibility in training will allow you to specialize, and add more training components as your needs change.

You will soon see how these features will make a difference for your swimming program, and your effectiveness as a swim instructor. Radically improved rates of progress will improve patron satisfaction, and give your program high visibility in the community.

Please explore the possibilities, begin your journey, challenge yourself to get the best from yourself and your students, and then adapt what works best to fit your needs. Welcome to Learn to Swim!

Acknowledgements

ABOUT THE AUTHORS

The primary work for the Learn to Swim program is the product of its author, Ronald Rhinehart. Mr. Rhinehart is a high school teacher and swim coach for the Albuquerque Public Schools in New Mexico. Ron wrote and developed the scripts for all nine swim journeys, as well as the Challenge program outline and instructional video. He also patterned the organization and administration of Learn to Swim after successful swim instruction programs he has directed over the past 25 years. Ron has been a Sr. Associate with Jeff Ellis & Associates since 1989.

The Exploration component was developed through the work of Jeff Ellis & Associates Director Jill White, along with Barbara Law, City of Tallahassee; and Marie Sheba, City of Kissimmee, FL. These individuals bring years of practical teaching experience, combined with a high sense of professionalism and a national perspective to the program.

The Adapted Aquatics manual is the work of E. Louise Priest. Ms. Priest is a nationally known authority is the area of aquatics for persons with disabilities, and a consultant in many other areas of aquatics. She is an author of several books and many articles, and has been Editor of the National Aquatics Journal, published by the Council for National Cooperation in Aquatics (CNCA). She has been a professional in the field of aquatics for thirty years, working with the YMCA, the American Red Cross, and CNCA. While on the staff of the American Red Cross, Ms. Priest wrote the text Adapted Aquatics, which was used extensively in the United States and Canada for more than 15 years, and in addition worked on American Red Cross Lifesaving and Lifeguarding materials. Ms. Priest is now a Director of Jeff Ellis & Associates, Inc.

ABOUT THE CONTRIBUTORS

In addition to Mr. Rhinehart, Sr. Associate, and Louise Priest, Director, we greatly appreciate and acknowledge the contributions of Sr. Associates Brenda (McVitty) Austin, Joe Minninger, Vera Solis, Richard Bleam, Chris Stuart; Associates Terri Adams, Scott Deisley, Andy Maurek, Chris Perry, Rafael Suarez, Joni Waggoner, Jim Wheeler, Rac Carroll; and Directors Carol Fick, Tabor Cowden, Jeremy Maloney, Norm Matzl, Mark and Mike Oostman. As Jeff Ellis & Associates, Inc. staff, these individuals were assigned supporting roles in developing the instructor's resource materials and provided perspective, information, and helpful review.

We also recognize the outstanding consultation provided by DoAnn Geiger and Rosemary Umenhofer. Both have coordinated large aquatic programs for the past thirty years with the YWCA, public schools, and community organizations in Rockford, Illinois. Their counsel and advice have proven invaluable to the project.

Lisa Mann and Glenn Pollack, City of Cape Coral, FL. have provided the Swim the Seven Seas component of the Fitness Challenge, and their efforts are greatly appreciated. In addition, Cape Coral Aquatics Supervisor Janis (Carley) Keim and Program Coordinator Mike Fischer, in addition to Dean Cerdan, Lee County Parks & Recreaton, have provided tremendous support and input into the process of the development of the Learn to Swim program components.

We wish to express our thanks to and acknowledge the contributions of Julian U. Stein and Susan Grosse. Both have given outstanding national leadership in the area of adapted physical education for many years, and provided extremely helpful review and critique of the adapted materials.

SPECIAL THANKS TO:

The facilities and Program Coordinators that implemented the Journey program at their facilities the first year and served as 'living laboratories' while the additional components were being developed: Sandy Baar, Boys and Girls Club of Sarasota, FL.; Carolyn Spencer, Faiview-Greenburgh Community Center, N.Y; Karen Kester, North Peninsula Recreation, Kenai, AK.; Bobbie Davis, Amarillo, TX; David Deal, City of Ft. Lauderdale, FL; Tom Carstens, Cary Park District, IL; Andy Maurek, Hyland Hills Parks & Recreation, CO.; Crystal Brown, Vandenberg Air Force Base, CA.; Zane Arters, Mesa Parks & Recreation, AZ.; Kelly Gentry, City of Pocatello, ID; Richard Jensen, City of Aurora Public Schools, CO.; Donna Best-Carlson, Lake Havasu Parks & Recreation,AZ.; David Landrum, Rupert Parks & Recreation, ID.; Edward Hartnett, Sunset Beach & Fitness, CO; Steve King, Ft. Richardson, AK.; Dan Maestas, Bernalillo County, AZ.; Nancy White, City of Rio Rancho, AZ; Gina VanBlockland, City of Gainesville, FL; Olivia Walters, Bastrop, TX.

Special appreciation also goes to the individuals who were a part of our initial review process. These include Gary and Andy Maurek of Hyland Hills Park and Recreation, as well as the focus group that met at the 1993 NRPA National Aquatic Conference. These individuals, from a wide variety of aquatic backgrounds and philosophies, provided insight, technique, and additional ideas that were valuable to the final development of the Journey books. The focus group included: Susie Boone, City of Lexington, KY.; Jim Ensign, Fox Valley Park District, IL.; Barbara Law and Patty Maloney, City of Tallahassee, FL.; Carolyn Mayberry, New Mexico State University, Las Cruces; Melody Medley of Medley Swim Systems, DE.; Larry Moscato, Dundee Township, IL.; and Allison Osinski of Aquatic Consulting Services, San Diego, CA.

Thanks also go to Fairfax County Park Authority, Fairfax, VA. and to the Council for National Cooperation in Aquatics, for the use of the photos in this manual. Most of the CNCA photos were taken in the IU Natatorium in Indianapolis, IN by photographer Greg McDermott. Additional photos were taken by Mr. Robbin White, with thanks to Sarasota Boys & Girls Club/Swim Florida swim team, Eldora Pool and Ice Center (EPIC)/Fort Collins Area Swim Team, and Mr. John Mattos, Head Coach, Colorado State University Swimming, for assistance and support.

Special thanks also go to Stephen J. Langendorfer, Ph.D., Bowling Green State University, and Tom Werts, Chairman, Florida HRS Aquatic Program Review Committee, for professional advice and insight which helped Learn to Swim evolve into a state of the art aquatic program.

Also helpful with the adapted program development were the constructive review and many suggestions of Bill Miller, of Columbus, OH and John Hunsucker of Houston, TX, and the mainstream teacher's perspective and suggestions provided by Bonnie Priest of Indianapolis, IN.

Special acknowledgement and thanks are expressed to Mr. Bill Markowski, National Safety Council, for the excellent production work in putting the Instructor Resource Manual together.

Finally, we wish to express our thanks to Neil Boot and Donna Siegfried of the National Safety Council; and Mr. Walter Johnson of the National Recreation and Parks Association. Their encouragement, endorsement, positive support, and leadership have enabled the Ellis team to coordinate the administrative protocols for the program, and make Learn to Swim possible.

Jeff Ellis - President   Jill White - Director, Learn to Swim
Jeff Ellis & Associates, Inc   Jeff Ellis & Associates, Inc.

Water Exploration

Water Exploration can be a wonderful experience for parent and child, if done safely and appropriately!

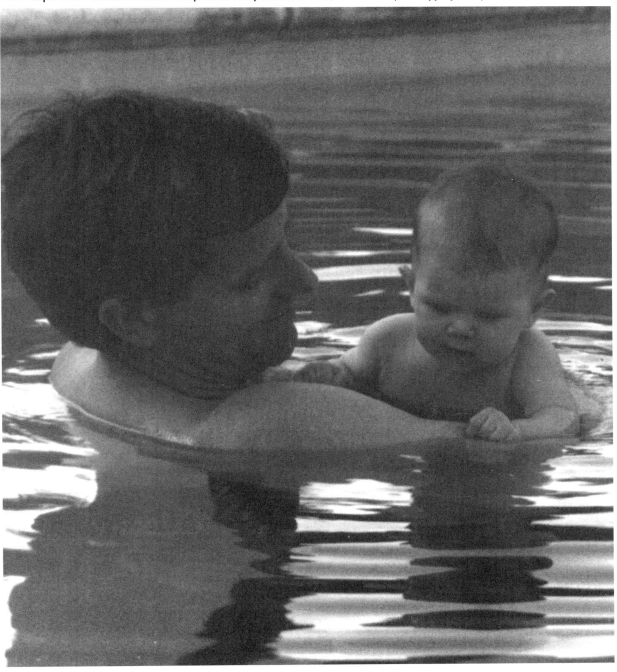

Children in the Exploration program are guided through the exploration activities by a parent or caregiver.

PROGRAM OVERVIEW

The National Safety Council Exploration Program, developed in conjunction with Jeff Ellis & Associates, is a community-based program for children ages 6 months - 3 years with a parent or caregiver. It is designed to be locally administered, with minimal expense, and with specific but easy to implement instructor training.

The National Safety Council Exploration program is one of a four part Learn-To-Swim series. The program is administered on a local level by a licensed Program Coordinator who is responsible for quality control, for the safety of participants, and for training instructors. Instructors conduct the classes under the guidance of the Program Coordinator, maintaining a maximum ratio of 12 children/parents per instructor. The Parent Handbook is used as a guide for instructors while conducting the program. The handbook is organized into a series of water safety topics and ideas for exploring body positions and movement in the water. CPR instruction, as well as strategies for managing an aquatic emergency are also included. The National Safety Council Exploration program is community-based in that the program coordinators administer the program, train instructors as needed, and oversee the scheduling and conducting of classes.

PROGRAM COORDINATORS

Program coordinators are trained and licensed by Jeff Ellis & Associates, Inc. Coordinators will be held accountable for maintaining the established standard of care for program safety, and facilities will be randomly and independently audited by Jeff Ellis & Associates to ensure compliance. Coordinators conduct instructor training according to the needs of the program, and are also responsible for regular in-service training of instructors.

INSTRUCTORS

Instructors may train for and be certified to teach the Exploration with the following prerequisites: Minimum age of 19, current CPR certification from a nationally recognized agency, experience in the care or teaching of young children or completion of child development courses, successful completion of the written test and practice teaching. The age prerequisite for instructor's may be lowered to 17 if the instructor is assisting with the class under the direct guidance of the Program Coordinator.

STUDENTS

Children in the Exploration Program are guided through the exploration activities by the parent of caregiver. The parent/caregiver is guided by the Exploration instructor in techniques for implementing the exploration water activities, in addition to the CPR and water safety components of the course.

INTRODUCTION

In the past ten years, infant and preschool swimming programs have seen tremendous growth, and the some locations, these classes are the most popular aquatic course. National agencies have developed guidelines for conducting such classes, and several excellent training programs for instructors have evolved.

For children under the age of five, drowning now outranks motor vehicle accidents as the single leading cause of injury death. Most aquatic professionals would agree that swimming instruction alone, especially for young children, cannot prevent drowning. It would seem, however, that if swimming programs for young children are so popular, these courses would provide a forum for educating parents about more practical forms of drowning prevention. According to National Safety Council statistics, the number of drownings in children under age five has remained virtually unchanged during the past ten years, despite the increase in parent/child swimming programs.

In examining reasons for this inconsistency, several interesting statistics related to childhood drownings were found:

- Ages one to two retain the highest rates for non-boating related drownings in the United States.
- Approximately fifty percent of all swimming pool drownings and near-drownings in children under age five occur in the child's own home, and the other fifty percent at the residence of a friend, relative, or neighbor.
- Only thirty percent of the drowning and near-drowning victims had on swim suits.
- **Two-thirds of the victims were "actively supervised" by one or more caregivers with a lapse in supervision prior to the incident of a few minutes at most.**
- Immersion times were usually brief, under five minutes.
- Forty-two percent of the victims died due to delay in CPR until EMS arrived because no one on site was trained in CPR.
- Likelihood that a child will survive with normal neurological status is largely determined by events that occur within ten minutes of the incident. For favorable outcome, brief immersion must be followed by prompt and effective resuscitation.

These statistics point to three major problems that contributed to the deaths of these children.
1. Ineffective drowning prevention strategies in the home.
2. Ineffective supervision and lack of understanding of what active supervision around water needs to be.
3. Lack of CPR skills or knowledge of what to do in an emergency.

In addition to providing a swimming program that is based on developmentally appropriate practices and follows all national guidelines, the National Safety Council Water Exploration program seeks to reduce the number of drownings of young children. The instructional format of the program is based around sound drowning prevention practices that are aggressive and active. This goal will be accomplished by:

- providing parents or caregivers with a practical and easy to use handbook. When supplemented with instructor reinforcement during class, the handbook will allow immediate implementation of drowning prevention strategies.
- implementing the "10/20 Rule" at the family level. This rule has become the standard of care for professional pool and waterpark lifeguards and has revolutionized the ability to measure lifeguard attentiveness and ability to recognized an aquatic emergency early. A parent or caregiver's understanding of what active supervision around water should be is open to wide interpretation unless there is a measurable standard from which behavior can be measured. The 10/20 Rule provides this standard.
- including training in basic emergency plan and CPR skills training as part of the course.

We welcome you to our family as a Water Exploration Instructor, and together let's make a significant impact in saving the lives of children!

Jeffrey L. Ellis - President • Jeff Ellis & Associates, Inc.
International Aquatic Safety Consultants
Training Agency for the National Safety Council Learn-To-Swim Program

OBJECTIVES AND CONTENT

Objectives of the course:

1.) Provide parents or caregivers with drowning prevention strategies that are practical and make sense.
2.) Provide a standard for measuring supervision of young children around water.
3.) Provide education on how to handle an aquatic emergency to improve the chances of survival.
4.) Provide information on how to perform rescue breathing/CPR.
5.) Provide a wide variety of water activities that are developmentally appropriate so that parents can explore the water in an enjoyable and safe manner with their children.
6.) Provide guidelines for developing good body position and movement skills that will prepare children for the development of correct swimming stroke skills as they get older.

Skills/Course content:

- The Water Exploration Program
- Swimming Lesson Safety
- Swish The Fish
- The 10/20 Rule
- Water Safety In The Home
    - Home Pool Safety Checklist
    - Home Pool Rules
    - In Case of An Emergency
    - Emergency Plan
- CPR
    - Checking responsiveness
    - Calling for help/activating EMS
    - Opening the airway/airway management
    - Look, listen, and feel
    - Two slow breaths
    - Checking pulse
    - Rescue breathing - child and infant
    - Foreign body airway obstruction, child and infant
    - CPR compressions - child and infant
- Water Safety on Vacation
- Exploring Body Positions
    - Front
    - Vertical
    - Back
    - Side
    - Changing positions
    - Games and activities
- Exploring Movement
    - Kicking
    - Pulling
    - Combination

The water should be explored in an enjoyable and safe manner.

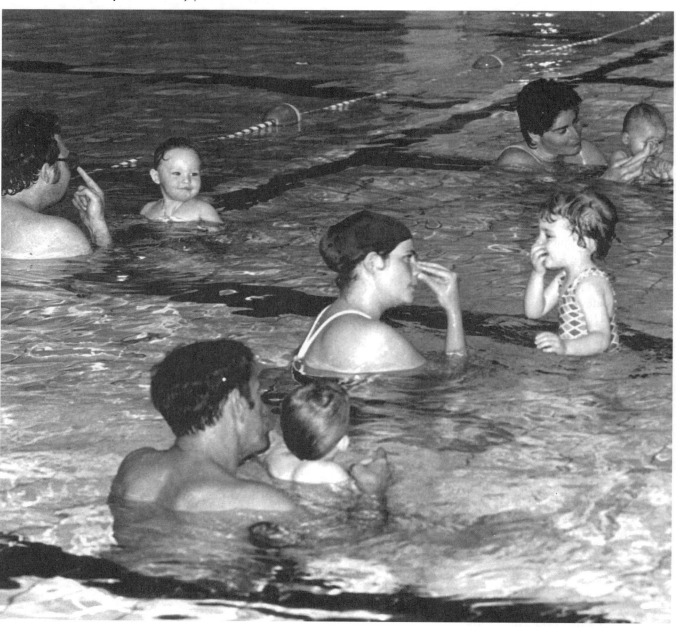

Each child will work at a different developmental level unique to that child.

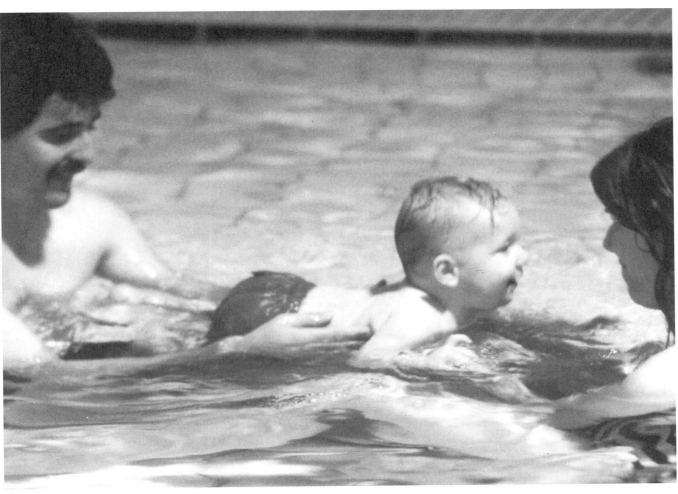

DESIGN OF LEARNING ACTIVITIES

- Small children will be happier if they are active.

- Be concise in your descriptions to parents/caregivers. Use the Parent Handbook as a guide for your lessons, and expand on the information. Ideas are presented in the Instructor Manual.

- New skills should be introduced, practiced for a short time, evaluated individually or in small groups, and repeated at each subsequent class.

- Competency should not be expected until the skill has been practiced in several classes. Parents should have a general knowledge of the "game plan" for each class. This will help the parents feel more comfortable and confident and they will not be worrying about "what's next?".

- Parents/caregivers should be made aware of the importance of attending all classes, being on time, and staying until the end of each class. If a child needs to be removed from the water before class is over, the parent/caregiver and child should watch from deck if possible.

- Information should be provided on the first class day (or during a pre-course orientation) regarding your facility policies and procedures. These policies might include: clothing restrictions, sign-in, potty training, older siblings attending class, weather/cancellation, etc.

- It is essential that all adult participants understand that each child will be working at a different developmental level that is unique to that child. Broad developmental guidelines for different age categories will be presented, but each child may perform skills at a different time or level of competency.

- Encourage parents to observe the differences in the way skills are presented and performed for different developmental levels. In this way, a parent will have the skills necessary to work with a child as the developmental level changes from infant, to toddler, to preschooler.

- Encourage adults to try everything. If a parent/caregiver is unable to perform some skills, or is frightened, suggest that another trusted adult familiar to the child attends to assist.

- It is important for all participants to recognize the end of class. Everyone should exit the pool area at the same time, with the instructor the last person off the deck to ensure the no one wanders back.

Water exploration is fun!

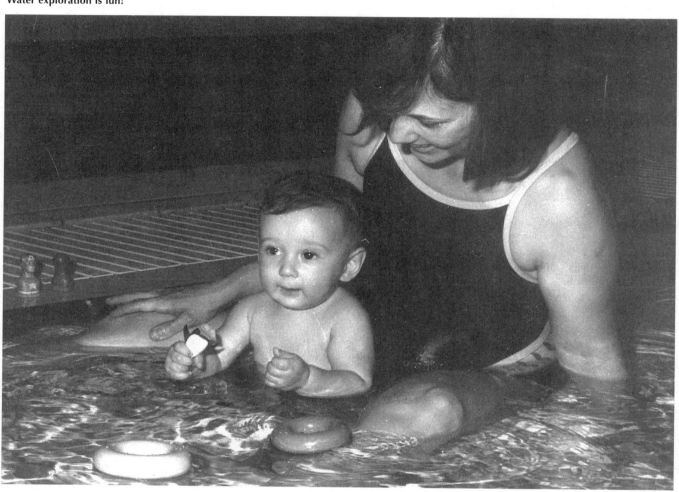

USING THE PARENT HANDBOOK

The parent handbook is an integral part of the National Safety Council Water Exploration program. Each parent or caregiver should be provided with a handbook the first day of class.

The Parent Handbook is designed to:
- **supplement the information you will present in class.**
- **provide information the parent/caregiver can use to reinforce skills after the course is over.**
- **give the parent/caregiver practical handouts that can be posted in the home.**
- **provide the framework for the Exploration curriculum.**

Encourage parents/caregivers to use the handbook frequently, and to take advantage of the practical manner in which the information is presented.

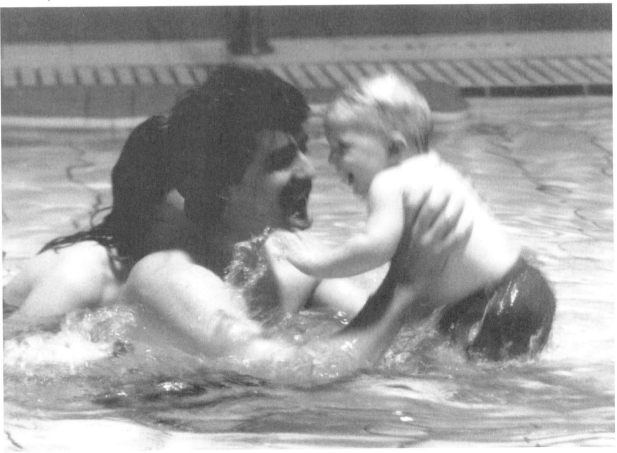

INSTRUCTOR'S PARENT HANDBOOK RESOURCE GUIDE

- The Water Exploration Program
- Swimming Lesson Safety
- Swish The Fish
- The 10/20 Rule
- Water Safety In The Home
- Home Pool Safety Checklist
- Home Pool Rules
- In Case Of An Emergency
- Water Safety On Vacation
- Exploring Body Positions
- Exploring Movement
- CPR

The pages that follow duplicate the text information in the Parent Handbook. Additional comments and explanation, along with photos, are provided so that you can effectively present these topics to the parents in your Exploration classes.

THE WATER EXPLORATION PROGRAM

Goals of the Exploration Program:

1) Provide drowning prevention strategies to parents that are practical and make sense.
2) Provide a standard for measuring supervision of young children around the water.
3) Provide education on how to handle an aquatic emergency.
4) Provide information on how to perform rescue breathing/CPR.
5) Provide a wide variety of water activities that are developmentally appropriate so that parents can explore the water in an enjoyable and safe manner with their children.
6) Provide guidelines for developing good body positions and movement skills that will prepare children for development of correct swimming stroke skills.

Welcome to the National Safety Council Water Exploration Program! You are about to explore a wide variety of water activities with your child through one of the most unique and state-of-the art programs available today.

Based on the research of Ellis & Associates, Inc.; International Aquatic Safety Consultants, the National Safety Council determined a need to establish a program to specifically address the issues of water safety and an appropriate introduction to the water environment for infants, toddlers, and preschoolers. The water exploration program is a result of these efforts. This program fully addresses the mission of the National Safety Council while enhancing the safety of this nation's children. The National Recreation and Parks Association has joined in this effort by endorsing this program.

This handbook is designed to be used in conjunction with the Water Exploration course taught by a certified instructor under the direction of a licensed program coordinator. It is a resource handbook only, and not a substitute for the instruction you will receive during classes. We encourage you to use this handbook to:
• post the pool rules if you have a home pool
• post the emergency plan near your pool phone
• review your CPR skills using the flow chart summary
• use the exploration pages as a guide when working with your child

Most of all, have fun and enjoy exploring the world of water with your child!

SWIMMING LESSON SAFETY

The National Safety Council Water Exploration Program follows the Guidelines for Swimming Programs for Children Under the Age of 3 set by the Council for National Cooperation in Aquatics (See Appendix D). In addition, the American Academy of Pediatrics recommends:

(See Appendix D)

These are guidelines set to provide a standard that all swimming programs conducted for young children should meet. Several states also have regulations for the certification and qualification of swim programs and instructors.

- When enrolling an infant or toddler in a water adjustment program, training should include the parent in the water with the child, and a certified swimming instructor.

- Instruction should be carried out by qualified instructors familiar with infant and child CPR techniques in properly maintained pools. Ask to see instructor's certifications.

REMEMBER...

- No child is ever "watersafe" or "drownproof", even with swimming skills.

    Prevention strategies, and maintaining the 10/20 Rule are the only methods of providing water safety!

- Practice water safety habits yourself. Be a good example.

    Children will follow what they see much more frequently than they will follow what they are told... especially if the two are different!

- Work with your child in water that is at least 78 degrees. Get out of the water and get dry at the first signs of chill such as shivering or blue lips.

    Being cold and uncomfortable is a big reason why many children cry when they are in the water. Children (and adults) don't have fun or learn effectively if the water and/or air are cold.

- Be aware of the amount of water your child is swallowing.
    Remove your child from the water at the first signs of a tight or bloated stomach.

    A child who swallows excessive amounts of water (or any fluid) too quickly can upset the electrolyte balance that regulates bodily functions. Actual occurrences are very rare, but the potential does exist if a child is "drinking" large amounts of water during the session.

- Your child should wear snug, tight fitting "training" type pants in the water, not diapers.

    Diapers weigh a child down, and are not effective at keeping urine and/or bowel movements from leaking into the water. Proper chlorination of the pool will eliminate any urine quickly, but special precautions need to be taken if any bowel movement enters the water. Instructors should be notified immediately if this occurs, and will follow proper procedure for the facility.

SWISH THE FISH

The Journey One book from the National Safety Council Learn to Swim Journey Series will be a great resource to use with 2 ½ - 3 year olds.

Encourage parents to purchase the books, and to do the activities with their children!

Introducing...the National Safety Council's official water safety mascot, Swish The Fish.
Swish will be introduced to you and your child in some of the exploration and water safety activities you will enjoy during your water exploration course.

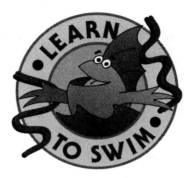

Once your child is ready for more formalized instruction (in a small group with a certified instructor) it will be Swish who will guide the learning journeys and adventures. The Learn-To-Swim Journey program will be the next step in your child's swimming development.

The Journey series is an innovative program designed for children ages 4-7. Each child receives a colorful storybook that captures the imagination as Swish and his friends experience all kinds of adventures and learn swimming skills at the same time.

Learning swimming skills becomes fun, and progress is rapid. Ask your Learn-To-Swim Program Coordinator about this, and other National Safety Council programs that your facility may offer.

THE 10/20 PROTECTION RULE

The 10/20 Rule is a standard by which you should measure all of your activities anytime you are around water. This rule has become the "standard of care" for professional pool and waterpark lifeguards, and has been responsible for reducing the number of drownings that occur every year in this country. Now you can make the difference, too!

Data from over 60,000 documented rescues prove that managing an aquatic emergency early, within the first 30 seconds, can prevent an incident from resulting in a drowning.

You should always be able to:
- See an emergency happen within the FIRST 10 SECONDS
  AND
- Be able to respond and give care within the NEXT 20 SECONDS

- Use this standard to question yourself: If I
  answer the phone...
  answer the door...
  check on the baby...
  read my book...
  mow the lawn...
  cook...
  watch TV...
  talk to a friend...

will I be able to see an emergency in the pool within 10 seconds and get to it within 20 seconds??????????????

The 10/20 Rule gives a measurable standard, or an accountability to supervision around water.

Make the 10/20 Rule a household word!!!

WATER SAFETY IN THE HOME

Even if the parents in your class do not have a home pool, the same water safety guidelines apply near any body of water. Reinforce that any parent will need to understand these guidelines whenever near a hotel, country club, condo, friend's or relative's pool.

- **Complete the Home Pool Safety Checklist often.**
  Make sure your pool and pool area are safe.
- **CONSTANT adult supervision of children.**
  Even a momentary lapse is supervision in the bathtub or pool can result in a tragedy. Never assume someone else is watching your child. If your child is missing, go to the edge of the pool and look in first. Maintain the 10/20 Rule!
  Continually reinforce the purpose of the 10/20 Rule.
- **Have (and practice) a family emergency plan**
  Everyone that uses the pool should know what to do.
  Demonstrate how to practice the Emergency Plan, and encourage families to practice it often.
- **Know CPR.**
  Seconds count in a drowning emergency, and the minutes it could take for EMT's to arrive could be the difference between recovery, brain damage, or death.
  Reinforce that CPR skills are easy to learn, and if practiced often, easy to remember. Encourage use of the CPR handout.
- **Keep a portable phone poolside.**
  Post the Emergency Plan Checklist near the phone.
- **Empty any container that will hold water.**
  This includes items such as buckets, inflatable pools, fountains, or aquariums that cannot be secured.
  Empty ANY container that a small child could get into, including bathtubs!
- **Use multiple barriers around the backyard pool.**
  Familiarize guests and pool users with barriers and gates to insure proper use. Always latch properly!
  The more barriers between the house and the pool, the more protection. Latches must be out of children's reach and be securely latched EVERY TIME after use.
- **Teach children water safety skills.**
  Children should be taught safety around the pool as well as how to swim.
  Reinforce that no child (or adult) is ever water safe, even with swimming skills.
- **Post pool rules.**
  Let swimmers know what they can and cannot do. Do not allow any activities that could lead to injuries. Make sure adults always set a good example.
  Encourage use of the Pool Rules handout. Suggest laminating it and posting it in a visible spot near the pool.
- **The pool deck should not be a "play area".**
  Most drownings and submersion injuries happen to individuals who did not intend to get wet.
  Instruct parents to tell their children to never enter the water to retrieve a toy.
- **Allow diving in water depth of at least 8 feet only.**
  Allow jumping only unless your water is deeper than 8 feet.
  Spinal injury is a real danger in shallow home pools. NO DIVING!
- **No swimming during electrical storms.**
  Exit the pool area at the first sign of approaching bad weather.
  Wait at least 30 minutes after the last lightning before re-entry.
  Lightning can also occur away, or ahead of, storm clouds. Whenever there is any threat of bad weather, stay out of the pool and pool area.
- **Have rescue equipment within reach.**
  Practice using equipment before an emergency happens.
  Examples would include poles, rope, ring buoy, rescue tube, or any reaching or throwing device that would float.

HOME POOL SAFETY CHECKLIST

❐ **More than one barrier that guards against unsupervised access from all sides.**
The house and doors going directly from the house to the pool area should not be considered a barrier.

❐ **Gates and doors ALWAYS latched or locked.**
An unlocked or broken gate or latch is like having nothing at all.

❐ **Routine checks to see that locks are functional.**
Make sure any person who will lock a latch knows how to do it.

❐ **Pool covers used according to manufacturer's directions.**
❐ **Pool covers removed completely when pool is in use.**
Never allow playing on or under the pool covers.

❐ **Fencing or landscaping does not block pool view.**
You must have a clear view of the pool area at all times.

❐ **Deep and shallow areas are clearly marked.**
❐ **Buoyed line separates shallow and deep end.**
A floating line is a visible feature that can show were deep water starts.

❐ **Rescue equipment is easily accessible such as a ring buoy, pole, throwing line, rescue tube, etc..**
Hang rescue equipment from a fence, or on a wall.

❐ **A clearly marked and well-stocked first aid kit is available.**
At the minimum, a first aid kit should contain latex gloves, resuscitation mask, Band-Aids, gauze, waterproof tape, ice pack.

❐ **Pool rules are established, posted, and enforced.**
Be consistent in enforcing rules, and make sure every guest knows what the rules are.

❐ **A phone is available in or near the pool area.**
❐ **Emergency instructions are posted near the phone.**
Post the emergency plan near each phone. If the phone is a cordless, make sure it is charged.
Family members and guests should know where the emergency plan is posted.

❐ **Family members know CPR.**
CPR skills should be reviewed and practiced often. Post the CPR summary chart in a visible location.

❐ **Water is clean and clear.**
Test water daily, and maintain proper water balance. If you cannot see the bottom of the pool clearly, do not allow swimmers in the water. Cloudy water is not clean, and prevents seeing a body on the bottom.

❐ **Pool chemicals and testing kit are stored in a locked area that is cool, and well-ventilated.**
Make sure pool chemicals are stored away from access by children. Post the Poison Control numbers on the Emergency Plan sheet that will be near your phone.

❐ **Water safety and swimming instruction are provided for all family members.**
All swimming instruction should be developmentally appropriate for the age and ability of each family member. All swimming instruction should also include personal safety and basic rescue/emergency skills. Swimming skills are lifetime skills.

ALWAYS MAINTAIN THE 10/20 RULE

Home Pool Rules

Encourage parents to laminate this sheet and post in a visible location near the home pool.

Post these rules in a visible spot, and review them with all family members and guests.

- **An adult must be designated to lifeguard when anyone is in the pool area.**
  Don't assume someone else is watching ...have a "designated pair of eyes".

- **No running.**
  The most common cause of accidents around a pool!

- **No pushing, dunking, or jumping on others.**

- **No glass around the pool.**

- **Dive into water only when it is 8 feet deep or deeper.**
  Shallow water presents a risk of spinal injury if entry is head first.

- **No swimming during thunder or lightning, or if a storm is approaching.**
  Lightning can come out of clouds ahead of a storm.

- **No breath holding contests.**
  Excessive breath holding can cause unexpected black-outs.

- **No swimming if under the influence of alcohol.**

- **Close the gate or secure the area when leaving.**

- **Know where rescue equipment is kept, and how to use it.**

- **Call 911 (or your local number) in an emergency.**

IN CASE OF AN EMERGENCY

1) Yell for help, and remove child from the pool.
2) **If you are alone:**
   - Check A,B,C's (Airway, Breathing, Circulation)
   - If the child is not breathing, perform 1 minute of rescue breathing/CPR.
   - Then call 911 or your local emergency number.

   If you are not alone:
   - Check A,B,C's and begin rescue breathing/CPR.
   - Direct another individual to call 911 or your local emergency number.

EMERGENCY PHONE NUMBERS

Emergency Number -   911

Doctor   _____

Hospital
Emergency   _____

Poison Control
Center   _____

EMERGENCY PHONE PROCEDURES

1) Dial emergency number.
2) Slowly and distinctly give your:

Name   _____

Location   _____

Phone Number   _____

3. Tell what happened, how many people need help, and the approximate ages of the victim(s).
4. Tell the emergency operator the condition of the victims. The most important information is whether or not the victim is breathing, or has a pulse, and what the skin color is.
5. **DO NOT HANG UP** until directed to do so by the emergency operator.
6. If possible, send someone to the front of the house to meet the ambulance and direct the EMS crew to the scene.

POST THIS BESIDE YOUR POOL AREA PHONE

1. Remind parents that if their child is missing, go to the EDGE of the pool FIRST, where the entire area can been seen, and look in.

2. The procedures are different for a child or an adult because the emergency care needs are a little different. An adult needs the immediate care that EMS can provide, and the ambulance needs to get there as soon as possible. A child, however, needs the first critical minutes of oxygen and rescue breathing /CPR should be supplied for that first critical minute before calling EMS if you are alone.

3. Write this information in ahead of time in case someone is responding to an emergency that is not a family member.

1. **Use rescue equipment. Do not enter the water, especially if you do not know how to swim.**

   Know your local emergency number, and usual response time.

2. **Remain calm so that you can communicate the information needed and help can be sent quickly.**

Make copies of this form if you have several phones in your house.

WATER SAFETY ON VACATION

Don't take a vacation from safety rules!

Reinforce 100% supervision and the importance of maintaining the 10/20 Rule.

• Scope out the pool before you swim.
  Is the water clean and clear? Where is the deep end? Where is the rescue equipment and how is it used?
  Is a lifeguard on duty? Where is the phone, and can you dial out directly?

• Never allow children to swim unsupervised in a hotel/motel pool.
  Never assume someone else is watching your child. Maintain the 10/20 Rule!

• Enforce the same safety rules you use at home.
  Consistency is a key ingredient with children.

• If you are planning boating activities be sure to take along a Coast Guard approved life jacket for each person.
  In many states, the law requires children to wear life jackets at all times in a boat. Also bring along other items that float, such as coolers, cushions, etc.

  Demonstrate use of a life jacket. Provide examples of different types of life jackets and show how to read the Coast Guard Approved labels and choose the right size. Demonstrate how to put on a life jacket in the water. Demonstrate other items that float and how these items can be used, such as a seat cushion, cooler, etc.

• Never allow children to swim, boat, or play around docks without adult supervision.
  Young children and weak swimmers should always wear a life jacket that is Coast Guard approved when near water.

• Know what is in, and under an open water area.
  Find out about hazards such as marine life, parasites, currents, drop-offs, very cold water, or submerged objects.
  Enter all unfamiliar water feet first (no diving) and caution children to avoid swallowing lake, river, or pond water.

  Encourage parents to find out first aid procedures for marine life that might be encountered such as stingrays or jellyfish.
  Fresh water parasites and bacteria can cause severe illness, so urge parents to be sure that the water is safe before allowing swimming. These organisms enter by swallowing water or through any body opening such as the ears.

• If the water area is shared by boats, be visible.
  Have your child wear a bright colored swim cap, stay close to shore, and actively watch for boats.

  Urge parents to allow swimming only in an area that is roped or buoyed, away from boat traffic. Remind parents that swimmers will be able to see boats much better than boats can see swimmers.

• Know what to do if your child falls in a river.
  Go downstream immediately to position yourself to help.

  Describe how a current will carry a child quickly away from the point of entry, and getting in at the place where the child fell in will put the rescuer behind and out of reach of the child.

EXPLORING BODY POSITIONS

Correct body positions will provide the framework for advanced swimming skills as your child gets older. Infants, toddlers, and pre-schoolers need to experience a variety of body positions and body position changes.

In working on body positions with your child:
- work on skills appropriate for their development. Use the summary on the following page as a guide.
- explore as many different positions as possible.
- combine body positions with movement.
- allow the water to provide most of the support - your role is to balance.

Getting In and Holding Your Child

Infants:
Have someone hand you your infant after you are in the water. Hold your infant away from your body as much as possible, and keep your shoulders submerged so that you are face to face.

Toddlers:
Sit with your toddler next to you on the side. Hold your toddler on the side with one hand as you enter the water and face him. Submerge to your shoulders, grasp him around the chest, and gently lift him into the water.

Preschool:
Encourage voluntary jumping or entering the water unassisted. Reinforce that she must enter the water ONLY with your permission.

It is your job to:
- maintain a safe learning environment
- balance
- lightly support

In working with:

Infants...you will control the body position

Toddlers...the body positions begin to be controlled by the child

Preschoolers...the body positions can be controlled, and the head position will will determine the body position. When the head is raised, the body becomes more vertical.

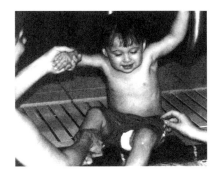
Adults should be in the water, and safely lift an infant into the pool.

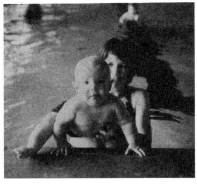
Encourage an independent but safe exit from the pool.

EXPLORING BODY POSITIONS
CONTINUED

Face to face, with eye contact, is important when exploring the water with an infant.

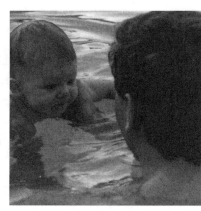

Experiment with different techniques to find what works best for each child.

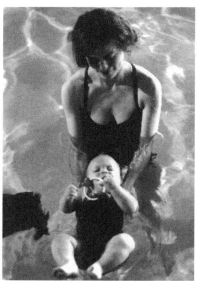

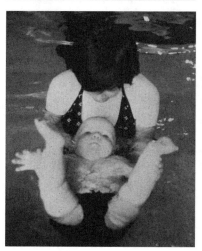

FRONT POSITION

Your shoulders submerged
Face-to-face
Your hands on child's chest, fingers spread and pointed toward feet
Thumbs over shoulders
Keep the child's body horizontal (on the surface)

Infants
Chin rests on heels of your hands

Toddlers
Will keep head up, your fingers can move off chest

Preschoolers
Use as little support as possible. An experienced child may submerge her head. Encourage straight legs and arms.

BACK POSITION

1) Hold your child with his back against your chest, cheek to cheek
Lower your bodies so that your child's head rests on your shoulder
Let his body float on the surface, lightly supported if needed.
2) Same as #1, except your child's head is off your shoulder, and moved to a position in the center of your chest. Hold the head.
3) Same as #2, except your child's body is moved away from your chest, and is being supported by the water. Hold the head only.

Infants
Move backwards. The water flow will help hold the body up.
Maintain this position as long as your infant is comfortable.

Toddlers
Perform this skill for short periods every time you are in the water.
Make sure the toddler's ears are in the water.

CHANGING POSITIONS

- Front to back • Back to front • Front to vertical
- Vertical to front • Back to vertical • Vertical to back
- Facing you to facing wall

Infants
Introduce a wide variety of body positions by placing your child slowly from one position to another.

Toddlers
Encourage your child to initiate a body position change. Assist with balance and support if needed.

Preschoolers
Encourage your child to initiate and perform a body position change. Assist as needed.

BODY POSITION GAMES AND ACTIVITIES

Toddlers enjoy games and songs as part of water exploration.

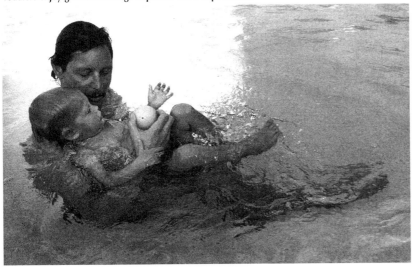

Independent purposeful play activities build confidence and understanding of the water.

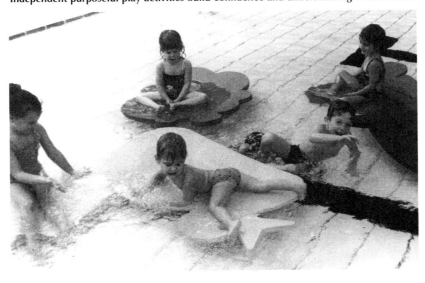

GAMES AND ACTIVITIES

- Sing "Rock-A-Bye-Baby" while rocking from side to side. Walk backwards as you sing.

- Humpty-Dumbty - child falls or jumps in from a sitting or standing position.

- Place toys on your child's chest while practicing back position skills.

- Imagination - Enter the pool like: crocodiles, marching soldiers, ducks with wings, elephants, etc.

- Twinkle, Twinkle - As your child is in a back position, sing Twinkle, Twinkle little star gently in her ear, while you both look for stars in the sky.

- Imagination - Be a leaf floating on a pond... a pancake that needs to be flipped over.

- Use arm floats (as a teaching aid only) to allow your child to experience various body positions.

- Assist your child while she rolls off the side, or off a raft. Follow up by initiating a body position/direction change back to the wall and safety.

Movement in the water is fun! The weightlessness of being in the water combined with the freedom of movement will provide an enjoyable experience as you and your child explore kicking, pulling, and gliding.

EXPLORING MOVEMENT

When working on movement skills:
- Always let your child set the pace. Keep your child motivated and she will want to move at a faster pace!
- Provide only as much support as your child needs to be balanced and have a good body position. Let the water and his movements do the rest!

SUBMERSION:

This course does not teach submersion skills. When your child is voluntarily submerging, or putting their face in the water, they are ready for formalized instruction with a certified instructor.

If your child should accidentally submerge or fall in the water, your reaction will be important. If you have maintained the 10/20 rule, you will be able to bring them to the surface immediately and prevent a life-threatening incident. A comforting hug, followed by getting back into the pool and continuing with your exploration will provide a positive experience rather than a negative experience that can be created if you over-react. Reinforce safety rules if the submersion was caused by a toddler or preschooler entering the water intentionally without permission.

Provide only as much support as is needed to provide balance for a good body position.

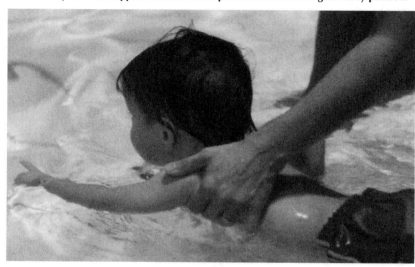

A child who is developmentally ready to submerge will experiment independently, and enjoy the experience.

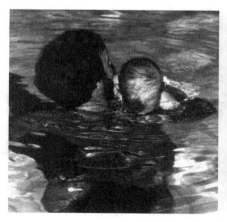
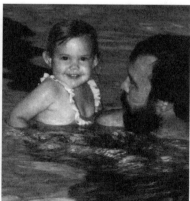

EXPLORING MOVEMENT - CONTINUED

Kicking techniques can be introduced by the parent physically moving the legs in the correct movement pattern.

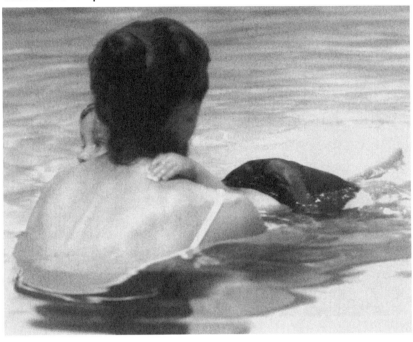

Always encourage independent movement, but be there to help!

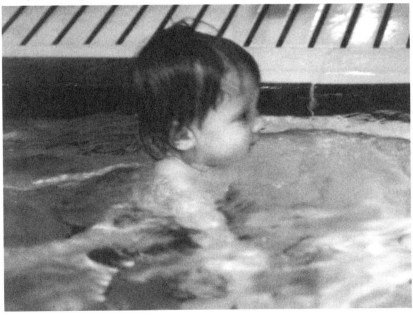

KICKING
- Movement is from the hips, with only a slight knee bend.
- Toes should be pointed.
- Kick is just below the surface... just to make a small splash
- Have your child face you and hold around your neck while you move their legs in the proper pattern.
- Use verbal cues such as "kick, kick, kick, kick..."
- Concentrate on pushing the water up toward the surface, rather than kicking it down toward the bottom.
- Kick in all body positions. Experiment with big kicks, little kicks, fast kicks, slow kicks.

Infant
Infrequent, voluntary leg movements may develop into propulsive kicking actions that resemble pedaling, running, or a frog kick. You will need to physically move the infant's legs in the correct kicking pattern.

Toddler
Pedaling action may change to simple flutter kick or frog kick action. You will still need to perform the correct kicking movements with physical manipulation.

Preschooler
Effectiveness of kick depends on body position. Your child will be able to control leg positions. Emphasize the "up" portion of the kick, rather than the "down".

EXPLORING MOVEMENT - CONTINUED

PULLING, FINNING, AND SCULLING

Pull movements should be toward the feet.

Pull in all body positions.

Experiment with big pulls, little pulls, fast pulls, slow pulls.

Use verbal cues.

Infant
Infants will usually show little voluntary pulling or arm movements. Movement may develop into voluntary splashing or weak paddling. Pulling movements must be physically manipulated, using the whole arm.

Toddler
Paddling may develop into alternate pulling, and your toddler should pull or exhibit arm movement upon command. Most voluntary movement will be underwater.

Preschooler
Voluntary movement of the arms out of the water (recovery) and then back into the water (pull) become more effective. Concentrate on "big arms" rather than underwater pulls.

Combination Skills
Provide support and balance only as needed. Use verbal cues, "Kick and pull", "Kick and pull"...

Infant
Combination skills are not practical at this developmental stage.

Toddler
Use verbal cues while physically manipulating the kick or the pull. Explore movement in all body positions.

Preschooler
Encourage voluntary direction changes, focus on getting back to the wall for safety.

Moving between two adults is a good way for children to practice combination skills and get the feeling of independent movement.

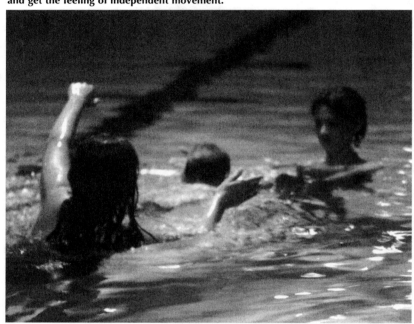

EXPLORING MOVEMENT GAMES & ACTIVITIES

A wide variety of experiences helps make learning fun.

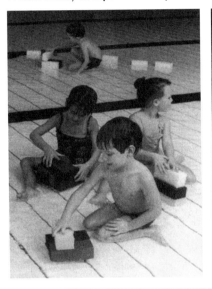
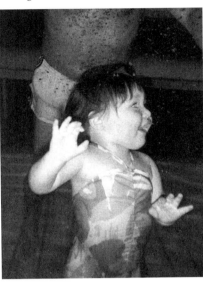
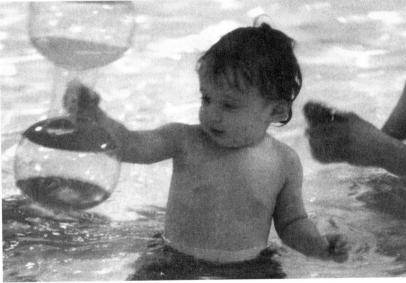

GAMES & ACTIVITIES

Piggy Back Ride - Back up against the side of the pool and have your child get on your back, putting his arms loosely around your neck. Proceed across the pool stooping with straight back while your child kicks her feet.

Red Light, Green Light - Skills are alternately started and stopped by the red light, green light commands.

Water Fountain - Have your child back float, and then kick to see how high the water can go, then how low. Do the same with splashing.

Loud & Quiet - Same as Water Fountain, but kick "loudly" then "quietly". Do the same with splashing.

Imagination - Have your child pretend she is a puppet, while you pattern their arms and legs; or a dog burying a bone. Make taffy. Mix a cake. Scoop ice cream.

Kick The Clouds - Support your child on the back. Have him stick his feet up in the air, first one at a time, then both together. What happens?

Motorboat - Same as Piggy Back, except start the motorboat engine by kicking. Speed up, slow down and stop by kicking fast, slow, or not at all.

Retrieve the Balls -Starting on one side, assist your child in moving toward and retrieving floating balls by pulling and kicking. Any floating object will work for this activity.

EMERGENCY CARE FOR CHOKING & CPR

EMERGENCY CARE FOR CHOKING

Many times, an infant, child or adult may be choking but conscious. Your quick efforts may be able to prevent a CPR emergency by removing the object that is blocking the airway before the victim loses consciousness.

Child or Adult

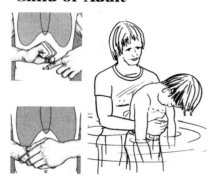

Infant

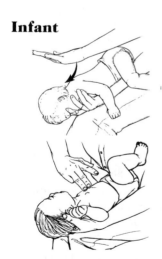

Repeat up to 5 back blows followed by up to 5 chest thrusts until:
• the infant becomes unconscious, or
• the object is expelled and the infant begins to breathe or coughs forcefully.

In an emergency, you can provide the care necessary to sustain life until the ambulance arrives. Artificial Respiration and CPR are easy to learn, and if practiced often, easy to perform.

Artificial Respiration (also called Rescue Breathing) is used if someone is not breathing on their own. It is the first step in any emergency...open the **Airway** and determine if the person is **Breathing**. If they are not, you will breathe for them. Next, you need to see if they have a pulse, or **Circulation**. If not, you will begin CPR. These are the A,B,C's of emergency care.

The first minutes are critical in any emergency. You must check the A,B,C's and act as quickly as possible.

You must also activate the EMS system (by calling 911 or your local emergency number so that an ambulance will be sent) as quickly as possible. They can provide the advanced life support that a non-breathing person needs.

If you are alone, and an infant or child needs rescue breathing or CPR:
• Yell for help. Someone may hear you and come to assist.
• Provide rescue breathing/CPR for one minute, then call 911 or your emergency number.

If you are not alone:
• Direct someone to call 911 or your emergency number immediately while you begin care. They can assist you after they have been released by the dispatcher.

Whenever possible, you should perform rescue breathing/CPR with a barrier such as a CPR pocket mask (available through medical supply companies) to protect yourself from disease transmission by bodily fluids.

Standing in a pool or shallow water
1. Stand behind the victim and wrap your arms around victim's waist.
2. Make a fist and place the thumb side of your fist against the victim's abdomen, below the rib cage and above the navel.
3. Grasp your fist with your other hand and press into the victim's abdomen with a quick upward thrust.

Victim lying on ground
1. Place victim on back. Turn face to one side to allow water to drain from mouth.
2. Facing victim, kneel astride victim's hips.
3. With one of your hands on top of the other, place the heel of your bottom hand on the abdomen below the rib cage and above the navel.
4. Use your body weight to press into the victim's abdomen with a quick upward thrust. Repeat until water no longer flows from the mouth.

This information is provided by the Heimlich Institute Foundation, Inc. and Jeff Ellis and Associates, Inc.

WATER EXPLORATION
SAMPLE COURSE OUTLINE

Sample 10 Lesson Course Session

Day 1
The Water Exploration Program
Swimming Lesson Safety
Getting in and holding your child
Parent/instructor roles

Day 2
Review
Swish The Fish introduction
The 10/20 Rule
Front position
Vertical position
Back position
CPR - checking responsiveness

Day 3
Review
Water Safety in the Home
Home pool checklist
Home pool rules
Side position
Changing positions
CPR-Opening the airway
     look, listen & feel

Day 4
Review
Emergency plan
CPR- calling for help, activating EMS
Kicking in all body positions

Day 5
Review
CPR - two slow breaths
     re-tilt if air does not go in
Pulling in all body positions

Day 6
Review
Rescue breathing - child
Rescue breathing-infant
Changing body positions using movement

Day 7
Review
Combination skills and exploration

Day 8
Review
Combination skills and exploration
CPR review

Day 9
Review
Working with another age child
Water safety on vacation
CPR-locating hand position
     compression rate and depth

Day 10
CPR skills practice
Course evaluation

Content of Each Lesson:
Review/orientation of day's activities.
Presentation of safety information.
Introduction of skill/activity.
Practice and individual evaluation.
Presentation of CPR information.

Off to a great start of life-long enjoyment of the water!

TEACHING CPR

The goal of the CPR portion of the Exploration program is to provide parents with familiarity of CPR so that in the event of an emergency, the parent would have a better chance of successful outcome by providing care until EMS arrives. There is no certification provided.

The CPR information in the Learn to Swim Exploration program is divided into two categories: CPR for a non-aquatic emergency, and CPR for an aquatic immersion (near-drowning) incident. The near-drowning CPR protocol information is provided by Jeff Ellis & Associates, based on their recent research into the most effective methods of handling a non-breathing victim after an aquatic immersion. At present, current National Safety Council/JAMA guidelines do not include this specialized protocol.

The CPR portion of the Exploration program can be integrated into the course in any manner that works best for your facility. Facilities have had equal success combining the CPR instruction a few minutes at a time at the end of class, or devoting a separate time for CPR away from kids and the pool. However you choose to structure the instruction, follow these guidelines for best success:

- keep it simple. Remember that you are not providing a CPR certification, but practical, helpful skill instruction. CPR is not difficult to learn, or perform. Stick to the basics so that your instruction is clear and concise.

- practice. Use the CPR skill sheets to pair up the class participants, and let them go through the entire "scenario" of an emergency situation. Each time, the skill level and level of confidence will improve.

- demonstrate. Be sure that your skills are at a performance level appropriate for showing others. Pay particular attention to your hand, arm, and body positions.

- combine group instruction, group drills, and individualized instruction.

- emphasize the importance of having an emergency plan, and calling for EMS in the event of an emergency. Clearly outline the procedure for both a water immersion emergency (utilizing the Heimlich maneuver **BEFORE** beginning rescue breathing) , and a non-water emergency. Remember to stress that if the rescuer is the only person available to call for help, and the victim is an infant or child, the rescue breathing/CPR sequence should be started and continued for about one minute before leaving the scene to activate EMS.

TRANSITIONS

TRANSITIONS - TO BE USED AT THE BEGINNING AND/OR END OF CLASS WHEN YOU NEED STUDENTS ATTENTION.

HELLO EVERYBODY
Hello everybody, yes indeed, yes indeed, yes indeed
Hello everybody, yes indeed, yes indeed, my darling.
2. Splash your hands
3. Blow bubbles
4. Kick your feet
5. Good-bye

HAPPY DAY
(She'll be coming 'round the mountain)

If your happy to be swimming,
• clap your hands (clap 2 times)
• splash your arms
• kick your legs
• blow the bubbles
• wet your head

I'M A GREAT BIG WHALE
(I'm a little tea pot)

I'm a great big whale (arms splash)
Watch me swim   (arms circle)
Here is my blowhole (tap head)
Here are my fins   (flap arms)
See me flip my tail and go down (123under)
The I come up and "Whoosh!"
I blow   (blow bubbles)

IF YOU'RE HAPPY AND YOU KNOW IT
If you're happy and you know it splash your hands
       kick your feet
       blow some bubbles
       get your head wet
       pat your back
       jump up and down
If you're happy and you know it, then your face (or life) will surely show it, if you're happy and you know it . . .(improvise with words and actions pertinent to your class).

MOTORBOAT
Motorboat, motorboat, go so slow.
Motorboat, motorboat, go so fast.
Motorboat, motorboat, put on the gas!

SWIMMING SONG
(Froggy wen a 'courtin)

Legs to kicking up and down splish splash, splish splash
Legs to kicking up and down splish splash, splish splash
Up and down and all around splish splash, splish, splash
Arms go flying up and around
Up and down but do not pound
Noses go bobbing in and out
In and out, now they're all wet

Children go swimming, they're so good
They're so good.. the songs all done.

O I WISH I WERE
Oh, I wish I were a little blue bubble (repeat)
I go floaty, floaty around everybody's boaty
Oh, I wish I were a little blue bubble (float hands)
Oh, I wish I were spiney like a starfish

2. I'd go crawley, creepy, crawley over everybody's belly (hands splash self)

3. Hard little crab
   Crawl in the sand and be so grand (underwater)

4. Eight legged Octopus
   Slidey slidey over everybody's hidey (kick legs)

HEALTH & SAFETY

There are several health and safety considerations that must be followed in order to provide a program for young children that meets national guidelines, and provides the safest possible environment and experience for children, parent/caregivers, and instructors.
In conducting the National Safety Council Exploration program, follow these guidelines:

1.) Concern: Hyponatremia (water intoxication). Because of the small body size and large skin area-to-body weight ratio, water ingestion can produce symptoms of hyponatremia. While rare, instructors and parents need to watch for signs of : bloated stomach, irritability, crying, vomiting. Prevention measures include:
- no submersion when a child is crying.
- submersions of young children during initial learning and exploration stage should be brief (1 to 5 seconds) and limited to six per lesson. When a child demonstrated competent breath control, submersion can become longer and more frequent.
- Parent/caregivers will be instructed to watch for water ingestion and discourage children from "drinking the water".

2.) Concern: Giardia (a parasitic infection) Giardia comes from contaminated pool water, usually contaminated after a patron has defecated in the water. Good pool chemistry prevents it. Most facilities have guidelines for treating this situation. Prevention measures include:
- Make sure the pool water is maintained to health code standards.
- Advise the parent/caregiver to use tight fitting training type pants on the child, not diapers.
- Advise parents to immediately notify the instructor if a child has defecated in the water.

3.) Concern: Ear infections. The most common ear infection is swimmers ear, which is an inflammation of the skin of the outer ear canal. It occurs after frequent water activity when water remains in the war and traps bacteria. Prevention measures include:
- Advise the parent/caregiver to consult a family physician for advice.

4.) Concern: Disease and infection. Sick children, or children with open sores or infections should not participate in swimming sessions. It is not beneficial to the child, other class participants, or the instructor. Prevention measures include:
- Develop a policy that prevents ill children or children with open sores/infections from attending classes.

5.) Concern: Hypothermia (low body temperature). Young children can become chilled relatively quickly due to low body mass. In addition, children cannot enjoy the experience or learn effectively if chilled. Prevention measures include:
- Conduct classes in water temperature that is at least 82 degrees Fahrenheit, with air temperature three degrees warmer.
- For infants and very young children, maximum in-water class time will not exceed thirty minutes.
- Parents/caregivers will be instructed to remove the child from the water at signs of chill.

6.) Concern: meeting special needs. If a child has special needs or medical conditions, a letter from the child's physician should accompany the course registration form.

Journey Program

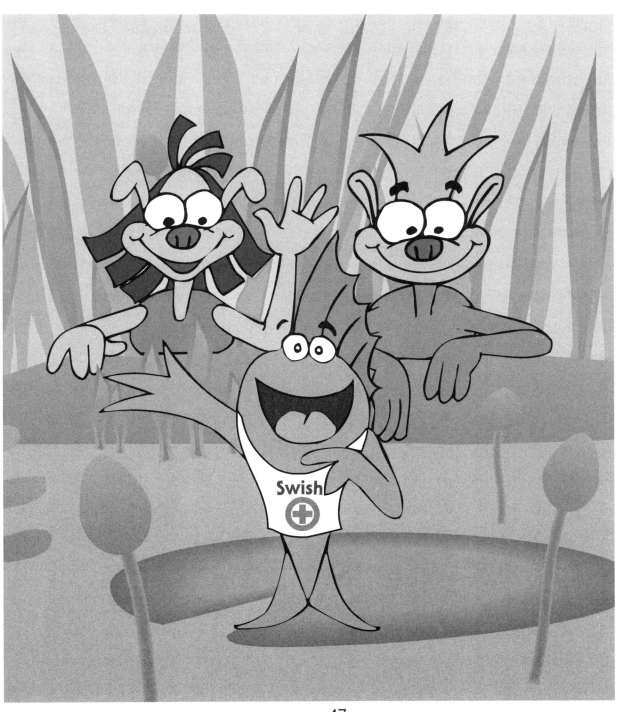

JOURNEY PROGRAM OVERVIEW

The National Safety Council Learn to Swim Journey Program, developed in conjunction with Ellis & Associates, is a community-based program for teaching 4 – 7 year olds to swim. It is designed to be locally administered, with minimal expense, and with minimal training time for instructors.

The National Safety Council Learn to Swim Journey Program is administered on the local level, by a program coordinator, who is responsible for quality control, for the safety of participants, and for training instructors. Instructors conduct the swimming classes under the guidance of the program coordinator, maintaining a ratio of 1 – 6 students per instructor. Instructors teach the class, using the stories and themes in the student booklets. The booklets are organized into a series of journeys, each with three adventures, in which the children learn aquatic movement and skills, demonstrated by various marine creatures. The bright, colorful booklets also contain progress checks and student activity pages which reinforce skills learned. The National Safety Council Learn to Swim Journey Program is community-based in that program coordinators administer the program, train instructors as needed, and oversee the scheduling and conducting of classes.

Program Coordinators
Program coordinators are trained and licensed by Ellis & Associates. Coordinators will be held accountable for maintaining the established standard of care and programs will be randomly and independently audited by Ellis & Associates to ensure compliance. Coordinators conduct instructor training according to their program needs.

Instructors
Instructors may train for and be certified to teach in any or all of the different journey levels. The prerequisites for training as an instructor are very simple: the candidate must be able to perform the skills in the level they wish to teach. Time involvement for instructor training is four hours per level.

Students
Students in the Learn to Swim Journey Program purchase the student booklets, each of which contains three adventures oriented around aquatic skills and marine life. These student booklets supply the themes for the different lessons. Instructors read the theme story to the students, and then guide the students in the water experiences associated with the adventure.

INTRODUCTION

Welcome to the National Safety Council *Learn to Swim Journey Program*, developed in conjunction with Jeff Ellis & Associates, Inc. This manual is intended to provide a general framework within which you can operate efficiently and enjoyably. The manual outlines the elements of effective teaching, characteristics of learners, and suggested teaching techniques for conducting and evaluating classes.

The program is creative, dynamic, and flexible.

The flexible guidelines provided in this manual emphasize the individualized nature of the learning process. Learning, especially for children, occurs in a variety of forms. Teaching methods, therefore, will vary with the course content, facility, and most of all with the students being taught. The National Safety Council Learn to Swim Program recognizes these realities and has developed a course that is creative, dynamic, and flexible. The Learn to Swim Program is designed to meet the needs of its participants and its instructors.

Your teaching plans must be efficient and organized.

Active participation by all students is the basis for the Learn to Swim Journey Program. Students do not learn by standing and watching. They learn by doing. It is the job of the creative instructor to actively involve all swimmers in whatever is taking place in the class. You will learn techniques that will help you be creative.

Your training does not end with this course.

To be effective, your teaching plans must also be efficient and organized. This manual will help you develop a systematic approach to planning, conducting, and evaluating your classes.

Your teaching style is uniquely yours.

Please remember that just as your students learn by doing, so do you! The best way for you to learn to teach is to teach. Therefore, your initial training course should be viewed as the first phase, or introduction, to continual development as you proceed through your career as a swim instructor. This resource manual will continue to be your guide.

The first six sections contain information that will help you understand the learning process. These topics are followed by resource pages for each adventure that will help you focus on the objectives for each adventure and give you guidelines and suggestions for planning your lessons. Other resource materials that you may find helpful can be found at the back of the manual in the appendices, and are referenced within the text.

Remember also that just as your students learn in different ways, so will you! Your teaching style is uniquely yours. You are about to embark upon your own journey, filled with the adventures of working with young learners. Have a great trip!

IDENTIFY STUDENT INFORMATION

To teach any class, you must have an understanding of the students: who and what they are, why they are in the class, and how much they already know about what you are teaching. It would be nice to know these things before class, but this is not always possible. Therefore, much of the information is gathered on the first day of class.

Find out the skill level of your students before instruction.

Student information helps the instructor judge what to teach and at what level the information must be presented. For example, a four-year-old beginning swimmer may not be able to progress as quickly or to learn as much as a seven-year-old swimmer. Likewise, older swimmers may have had unpleasant experiences in attempting some skills, and may be reluctant to continue. Therefore, it is necessary to determine the skill level of all beginning swimmers before the formal instruction begins.

In addition to determining skill level, it is necessary to understand that young learners possess some (if not all) of the following characteristics:

- Young learners are making a transition from being dependent on parents to being independent.
- Young learners respond differently to authority:
    some fight it, some flaunt it;
    some ignore it, some are frightened by it;
    some resent it, some crave it;
    some yield to it, some do not.
- Young learners may have a great deal of information based on experience.
- Most young learners experience discomfort when they are not allowed to move around.
- Young learners have established habits; when these habits are violated, learning may be difficult or impossible.
- Young learners are the products of the adults around them. These adults may be
    organized or disorganized,
    impatient or calm,
    aggressive or reticent,
    open or defensive,
    warm or aloof.

Not all people learn in the same way.

In young learners, these characteristics may change weekly, daily, or hourly.
- Most young learners have strong feelings about learning situations. These feelings are based on prior experiences, good or bad.

To help you deal with the many different responses young learners may have to your instruction, suggestions for dealing with the ten most common situations you may find yourself in follows.

The good instructor must learn as much as possible about the students being taught, and must try to develop positive feelings about learning how to swim. Not all people learn in the same way. Some must learn step-by-step, while others will be able to learn an entire skill at once. Some learn best in groups, while others learn better alone. However, all learners must feel that their learning is worthwhile. This can be achieved by recognizing the effort put forth in learning a skill, as well as the mastery of that skill.

Recognize effort as well as skill.

THEMED TEACHING

For years, Jeff Ellis & Associates, Inc. lifeguard auditors have observed young children in water play areas of large waterparks. When children are absorbed and enchanted with the games and characters found in the parks, they often downplay or do not notice the normally unpleasant experiences of getting water in their faces or up their noses.

Involved children learn while having fun.

By designing the National Safety Council Learn to Swim Journey Program to introduce each lesson with a story (theme-ing), we hope to provide the same sort of imaginative focus. It is called *teaching by deception*. If the students are occupied with stories about alligators, whales, seals, and otters, they will be less likely to worry about such things as getting their faces wet.

In addition, the students will be challenged to determine the best method of learning a particular skill, rather than simply copying the instructor. Using frequent references to the characters in the book and story line, students are asked questions that get them to think about the experience of performing a skill. For example, when teaching a recovery from a front or back float, a traditional method would involve telling the child to bend his or her knees and sit up. Using a facilitating method, the instructor asks the young learner, "Where do your feet need to go when you want to stand up?"

Such facilitating questions are designed to stimulate movement exploration or require a verbal answer that is not just a yes or no. Research with young learners has shown that this method not only keeps students more interested, but also that by adding language to tell about or describe a movement, they learn faster. This type of questioning keeps the learners' minds active, as well as their bodies.

Students who describe a movement learn faster.

DEALING WITH YOUNG CHILDREN IN LEARNING SITUATIONS

Ten Most Common Incidents	Suggested Actions
1. Child refuses to get into pool, or says no to everything	• Be firm but gentle • Make sure you are telling, not asking. This puts you in control and does not let the child have an opportunity to defy you. • Help the child get started—offer a special place on your back as lesson continues. • Distract or attempt another activity. • Make sure you have total group involvement. • Reward effort, no matter how small. • Use peer pressure and excitement of group to motivate.
2. Bullies others in group	• Catch behavior early. • Keep message simple and to the point. ("At the pool we use our arms to help us swim. We don't splash."). • Separate the child from the group, or distract with alternate activity.
3. Demands attention to the point it becomes disruptive	• Praise an effort, then be specific when it will be their turn again. • Give a special task. ("Let's both watch Jason kick. Can you tell me if his legs are straight?") • Be unpredictable so the child focuses on you, not himself/herself.
4. Withdrawn, won't interact	• Pair up in a short activity. • Reward effort, no matter how small. • Hold in arms for awhile, but don't say anything, and continue to teach. Occasionally say, "It's now your turn, let me see you try." • Look for anything that sparks interest, and use it to get the student involved.
5. Scared	Moderate fear • Provide distractions. • Involve in group. • Develop rapport and trust. • Be gentle but don't coddle. • Talk about fear. • Explain what is going to occur in lesson. • Give firmly stated positive suggestions.
5. Scared (cont.)	*Extreme fear* • Physical contact • Enlist help/support of parents. • Keep involved in group as much as possible – use peer pressure • Focus on skills that will build trust.
6. Cold	• Keep active and occupied. • Deflect comments about the cold. • Keep your own comments/discomfort to your self.

7. Asks or makes comments about drowning

- Use as a teachable moment for the entire group and to prevent further comments.
- Ask "What do you think drowning is?"
- Make statements such as "What we are here to do is to learn to swim and how to be safe around the water." "Children who swim with an adult watching do not drown" "What you learn will help keep you safe".
- Talk with the parent if there is continual concern.

8. Cries

- Distract.
- Physical contact, firm but gentle.
- Remove from sight of parent.
- Lots of talk to get distracted or total silence.
- Avoid bribing, making deals.

9. Temper tantrum

- Be firm but calm.
- Remove child from area if possible.
- Offer an activity as a transition to getting involved in the group again.

10. Won't stay put, runs to parent

- Ask parent to leave area.
- Sit with the child in your lap, or put child on your back.
- Distract, involve in group, – be unpredictable to spark interest.
- Praise when they do not run away.
- Put in a situation where child is dependent upon you (on your back, etc.)

OBJECTIVES AND CONTENT

Let's look now at how you will decide what you are going to present in a lesson, since you obviously cannot be all things to all people at all times.

Your input during in-service training is important.

In most cases, your program coordinator will present you with the adventures (courses) that you are to teach. There will be regularly scheduled in-service training during which you can discuss the appropriateness for your students of the skills being taught. Because you are the person directly dealing with the students, your input during the in-service training sessions is very important. If too many or too few skills have been chosen for the class, the situation will need to be communicated and corrected as soon as possible.

Objectives, goals, and outcomes must be carefully outlined — for the benefit of both the learner and the instructor. Lessons should not be treated like surprise parties, where students show up and see what happens. Objectives provide road maps or guides that help the learner and instructor know in which direction to move.

Course objective example: Develop floating skills.

There are two types of objectives that you will be using while teaching the National Safety Council Learn to Swim Program. The first is an adventure (course) objective. These objectives are listed at the top of each journey page in your instructor manual, and describe what the focus of the lesson will be. This type of objective also provides guidelines for the instructor in designing activities to help the learner move forward.

Learning objective example:

Swimmers will learn to stand up from a floating position.

The second type of objective is a learning objective, which indicates that some change is going to take place as a result of the instruction. Such objectives identify not what the instructor will be doing, but what the learner will be able to do as a result of the instruction. Learning objectives, no matter how carefully written, cannot specify or describe all the learning that may occur, because learning has a domino effect, and some learning causes more learning. However, if you specify certain learning objectives for a lesson, and they are met, then all concerned parties are satisfied.

The journey pages in this instructor manual contain several learning objectives for each journey. Use these objectives as your road map to help you design your lesson. Let these objectives be your servant, and not your master. How you achieve these objectives, and at what pace, are your responsibilities as an instructor. Be prepared to speed up or slow down as needed. The necessity of flexibility has already been discussed, be ready to modify your program to meet the needs of your students. As you use the objectives to begin designing your lesson, keep the following in mind:

Be prepared to be flexible.

- Don't try to cover too much in one lesson.
- Keep the lesson interesting and keep it moving.
- Make the participants feel some responsibility for their own learning.
- Make it fun to learn in your class.
- Know what you want the students to achieve and make it happen!

DESIGN OF LEARNING ACTIVITIES

What works for one may not work for another.

After setting your objectives and goals, it is time to design the learning activities you will provide for your students. You are completely free to plan and design your lessons in any way that works best for you, your facility, and your young learners. What method works for one may not work for another. If you have done your planning well, you took into consideration the characteristics of the people you are teaching, and you are well on your way to setting a positive learning climate.

However you construct your lesson plan, there are five major components which, under most conditions, should be a part of any lesson. This 5-step approach consists of

1. Set the climate for learning (physical and emotional).
2. Motivate.
3. Demonstrate.
4. Practice and facilitate.
5. Reinforce.

The order in which you perform these steps will vary according to your lesson plan. But, be sure you are using all five components. Let's look at each one more closely.

Setting the Learning Climate

The first few minutes of a lesson are important.

Successful swim lessons do not just happen. Setting the climate for learning begins with the first class and continues throughout the course. Similarly, the first few minutes of each lesson are extremely important. If the climate is conducive to learning, you will have no trouble filling your classes. If not, expect your enrollment to decrease. Preparing the physical environment is the first step in setting the learning climate. The appearance of the pool, instructor, and atmosphere in general all have an effect on student learning. Before each lesson begins, you need to prepare the physical environment. Set up a procedure for accomplishing this, keeping in mind the following:

Safety is our top priority.

- Safety is our top priority. Check your area for any safety hazards. Make sure a lifeguard is on duty. Check all equipment you plan to use to be sure it is safe and in proper working order. Review your Emergency Action Plan.

- Check the water quality, temperature, sun angles, and noise level. You may have to adapt your lesson plan if there are conditions in your teaching environment that you cannot control.

- What about you, the instructor? You are part of the learner's environment. Be sure that you look professional, and that you are emotionally ready to teach. Arrive on site with enough time to get all your materials and equipment organized, check your area for safety, and get ready to be fun and exciting!

Now that the physical climate is set and your students arrive what you do next can make or break your lessons. Setting the emotional climate is just as important as the physical one. The first few minutes of the lesson are crucial. If, during the first few minutes of the course, the atmosphere is pleasant and the presentation is interesting, then a positive attitude toward learning will prevail. If the first few minutes are seen as pointless, boring, or unpleasant, then a negative attitude is more likely to be formed. Here are some suggestions to help make your first few minutes positive ones.

If the first few minutes are seen as pointless, boring, or unpleasant, then a negative attitude is more likely to be formed. Here are some suggestions to help make your first few minutes positive ones.

Young swimmers need to feel they are welcome.

- Greet your students. Young swimmers need to feel that they are welcome in this strange new environment. Avoid herding large numbers of students from place to place on the first day of lessons. Learn the names of students and use them as soon as possible.

- Get everyone emotionally comfortable. Young swimmers' anxiety about a new learning environment should not be compounded by their getting into the water immediately. Sit everyone down and read the story for the lesson you will be teaching. Young learners will have been exposed to this learning situation, and will more easily transfer learning to the water when it becomes necessary.

- Begin developing group dynamics that will motivate, the students and allow you to maintain control of the group. Use peer pressure, excitement, unpredictable strategies to get the students moving and achieving immediately.

- Develop trust. Set up activities that force students to trust you, such as working in deep water the first activity of the lesson.

Motivation

This step in designing your learning activities gains attention and presents information. The initial motivation begins when you read the stories detailing the adventures of Swish the Fish and his friends Jonathan and Stacey. Next, you need to use the story theme to develop activities that will entice the students to want to try the skills in the water. Each story is designed to tempt the imagination of the young learner and introduce the skills that will be part of their lesson.

The adventures introduce the skills.

Demonstration

This step presents a given skill as it should be performed. For this step, the instructor must be able to successfully demonstrate the particular skill. When demonstrating a skill, use the following guidelines:

- Make sure your class is arranged so all students can see the skills being demonstrated.

- If your eyes will be off of your students while you demonstrate, make changes in your class organization to minimize risk.

- Give your students a task to do while watching your demonstration. For example, if you are demonstrating crawl stroke breathing, tell your students, "I am going to show you how to breathe. Where will my arm be when I take a breath?" After your demonstration, ask them to tell you what they observed. This technique can work for any part of any skill.

- Keep demonstrations short and specific to one skill.

Practice and Facilitate

This step allows the student to try the skill as presented by the instructor. During this step, the instructor may present parts of a skill, the entire skill, or appropriate combinations of steps needed to master a skill. Each adventure resource page in your instructor's manual contains several facilitating questions that you may find helpful to use in guiding your students during practice. Keep students moving with drills and activities that can be performed by more than student at a time.

Reinforce

This step allows the students to repeat a given skill and gives them feedback on their performance. At this point in the lesson, the instructor should place the individual skills into a meaningful scenario, which allows the students to appreciate the value of the learned skill.

Enthusiastic, positive comments combined with a specific suggestion for improving performance should be given after each student attempt

Reading Stories to Young Children

- Place yourself so you can see the book, and your students can also see. Holding the book off to one side and looking over your shoulder is one suggestion.
- Read the story, both silently and aloud to yourself several times before reading it to your students.
- Read to entertain! Put appropriate expression in your voice.
- Move the book around so all students can see the pictures before turning the page or closing the book.
- Smile and use facial expressions.
- If it is obvious that a child wants to make a comment during the story, allow it and use it as a teachable moment when you may be able to expand on an idea.
- Emphasize the end of a sentence. This helps you stay upbeat.
- Have fun!

Learn to Swim Journey Course Outline

Journey 1

Down under the Sea (adjustment to water)
- Movement in the water
- Breath holding
- Submersion of face
- Opening eyes
- Holding onto wall and bobbing

Alligator Alley (float/float with kick)
- Review all skills in previous lesson
- Stomach float and kick
- Begin back float
- Stomach float with kick to wall
- Stomach float with kick to instructor

Seal's Rock (beginner stroke/change directions)
- Fall/jump off slide
- Change directions, return to wall
- Begin pulling water
- Introduce sequence: float, kick, pull
- Cover distance of six feet
- Recover for air

Journey 2

Seaweed Patch (Freestyle)
- Arms in crawl motion
- Tap on head to time breathing, then assist breathing motion (place hand under chest to get up for air)
- Introduce side to side breathing
- Tread water

Otter's Cove (backstroke)
- Float and kick on back
- Roll over from back to front
- Begin sequence: float, kick, pull on back
- Push off on stomach, dive, float to surface, roll on back and move back to side

Tadpole Pool (breaststroke)
- Introduce breast stroke legs with aid
- Pull both arms while standing on bottom
- Introduce sequence: float, pull/breathe, kick, then glide
- Increase distance

Journey 3

Frog Pond (elementary backstroke)
- Review back float
- Introduce breast stroke on back
- Make a cross with arms
- Introduce sequence: kick/arms, then glide
- Increase distance

Dolphin's Den (butterfly)
- Double arm crawl
- Dolphin kick
- Kick with breath at end
- Introduce sequence: kick, pull, breathe
- Increase distance

Flounder Farm (sidestroke)
- Introduce body position on side
- Introduce arms separately with aid
- Introduce legs with aid
- Introduce sequence: pull, kick and glide]

INSTRUCTORS: Remember that the Journeys do not have to be taught or learned in any specific order.

For example, some students may master skills on the back before being able to have breath control.

Allow each student to work within the Journey level or adventure best suited to developmental needs and abilities.

INSTRUCTOR'S ADVENTURE RESOURCE GUIDE

1. Down under the Sea
2. Alligator Alley
3. Seal's Rock
4. Seaweed Patch
5. Otter's Cove
6. Tadpole Pool
7. Frog Pond
8. Dolphin's Den
9. Flounder Farm

Adventure Objectives

physical and mental adjustment to the water; lifeguard awareness

Learning Objectives

- Swimmers will become relaxed in the water.
- Swimmers will learn fundamentals of breath holding and exhaling on the surface.
- Swimmers will submerge face and use breath holding techniques under water.
- Swimmers will hold breath and open eyes under water.
- Swimmers will bob several times in a row, holding their breath and opening their eyes under the water, and exhaling through their nose to the surface.

Procedure

1. Read *Down under the Sea.*
2. Start journey by getting wet.
3. Next, wade in water and look for animals on the bottom. Animals should be the same as the ones mentioned in the story.
4. Have swimmers pick up animals from bottom.
5. Introduce breath holding at the surface. Inhale through mouth, exhale through nose.
6. Slowly, patiently have swimmers transfer skill to in-water use.
7. Have swimmers hold breath and open eyes while holding onto side of pool. Have them identify animals under water.
8. Place some animals in water deep enough that swimmer must place their faces in water to reach them.
9. Have swimmers get animals from the bottom.
10. When swimmers can pick up several animals in a row, have them move to the next journey.

DOWN under the SEA

As Swish the fish played his guitar, Stacey and Jonathan hummed along to the music. Swish looked like a flag waving underwater as he swiggled to the music they made together.

"Do you know that if you hum underwater," said Swish, "you can make a musical bubble noise?"

Jonathan and Stacey had never hummed underwater, but they liked the idea of making musical bubble noise. So they stepped into the water, first up to their knees, then up to their hips, then up to their chests. It felt great!

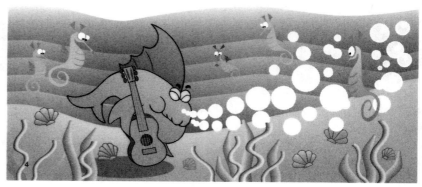

"Keep humming," said Swish, "and try to swiggle—you know, sort of swim-and-wiggle." They put their faces underwater and swiggled, but bobbed back up again.

"We got *wadder* up our noses," they said. "We'll just stand here and hum with our faces out of the water."

As they were humming along, a wave came up behind them, before Swish could warn them. "Are you all right?" asked Swish. "Did you get water up your noses?"

Stacey and Jonathan giggled. "We're fine. The hum kept bubbles blowing out of our noses and that kept the water from coming in. "Watch this!"

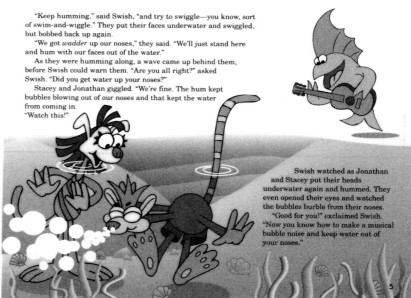

Swish watched as Jonathan and Stacey put their heads underwater again and hummed. They even opened their eyes and watched the bubbles burble from their noses.

"Good for you!" exclaimed Swish. "Now you know how to make a musical bubble noise and keep water out of your noses."

Instructor's Questions

1. Can you make humming music under water like Swish?
2. What do you think "swiggling" is like?
3. How does the water feel?
4. What does it feel like to hold your breath?
5. When you breathe out on land are there bubbles?
6. Are there bubbles in the water when you hold your breath?
7. When you breathe out under water, where do the bubbles come from?
8. What do you see under the water?
9. What animals can you pick up?

Teaching Tips

- Hold animals to control the depth they will reach.
- Use the stories and characters to create excitement.
- Avoid making a big deal about water in the eyes or ears.

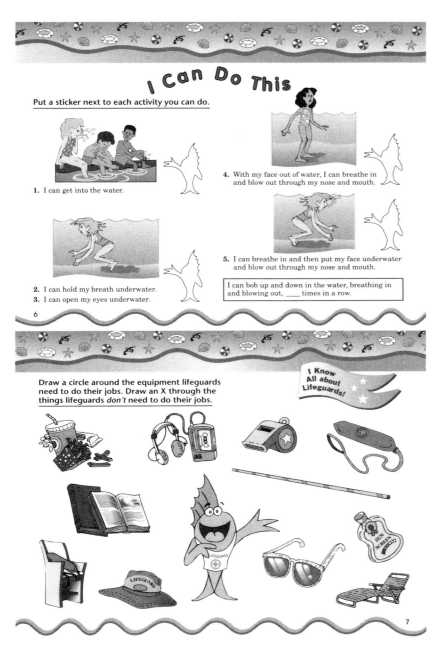

I Can Do This

Put a sticker next to each activity you can do.

1. I can get into the water.

2. I can hold my breath underwater.
3. I can open my eyes underwater.

4. With my face out of water, I can breathe in and blow out through my nose and mouth.

5. I can breathe in and then put my face underwater and blow out through my nose and mouth.

I can bob up and down in the water, breathing in and blowing out, ____ times in a row.

6

Draw a circle around the equipment lifeguards need to do their jobs. Draw an X through the things lifeguards *don't* need to do their jobs.

I Know All about Lifeguards!

7

Safety Considerations

- Make sure students can hold their breath on the surface before performing in the water.
- Watch for students that are so eager to please they will attempt anything, even if they or you are not ready.
- Never turn your back on your students.
- Keep yourself between your students and deep water.
- Always enter feet first in shallow water. Set a good example!
- Know your Emergency Action Plan.

65

Adventure Objectives

body position/floating; open water safety

Learning Objectives

- Swimmers will practice breath holding.
- Swimmers will learn about buoyancy.
- Swimmers will learn to relax while floating
- Swimmers will learn to stand from floating position.
- Swimmers will learn to straighten body while floating on stomach.
- Swimmers will begin to kick while floating on stomach.
- Swimmers will learn to use a kickboard.
- Swimmers will learn back float/back glide.
- Swimmers will kick on back.
- Swimmers will learn to recover to feet from a float.

Procedure

1. Read *Alligator Alley*.
2. Review breath holding by diving for animals.
3. Introduce jellyfish float, with knees under body.
4. Practice standing from jellyfish float.
5. From jellyfish float, straighten body.
6. Straighten body while standing, then fall forward and float.
7. Fall forward, float, and begin to kick legs.
8. Have swimmers hold breath, fall forward, float and kick a set distance.
9. When swimmers can kick a set distance to the instructor, move to the next adventure.
10. Introduce using a kickboard.
11. Introduce recovering from a back float.
12. Practice back float.
13. Practice back float, adding glide.
14. Practice back float, adding kick

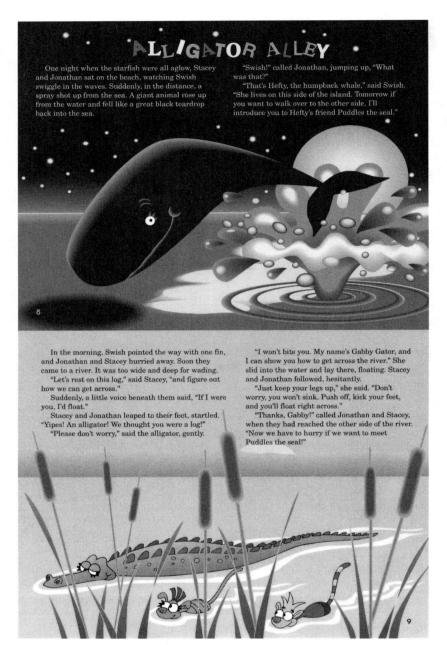

Instructor Questions

1. How does a jellyfish dangle its arms and legs?
2. How can you relax when you float on your stomach? What does Gabby look like when he floats? Does he swiggle when he floats?
3. How can your legs be a motor for your kickboard? Tell me about your knees and feet when you kick.
4. What would Gabby look like if he floated on his back?
5. How does Gabby glide across Alligator Alley on his stomach? On his back?
6. How can Gabby and you glide faster on your backs?
7. Where do your feet need to go when you want to stand up?

66

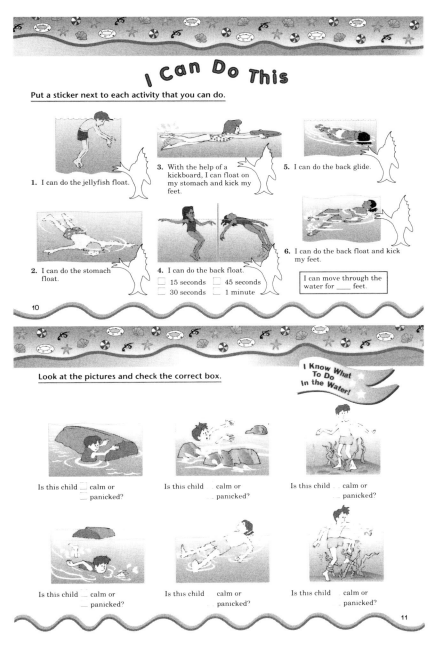

Teaching Tips

- Relax arms while holding kickboard, but hold with straight arms, elbows locked.
- Upper back should be on water surface in jellyfish float. Place hands on knees and look at both at bottom to control extra movement of arms and legs.
- Supply only as much balance and support as needed, at head or shoulders, not around middle.
- Let the student feel the support of the water, not you.

I Can Do This

Put a sticker next to each activity that you can do.

1. I can do the jellyfish float.
2. I can do the stomach float.
3. With the help of a kickboard, I can float on my stomach and kick my feet.
4. I can do the back float.
   - ☐ 15 seconds   ☐ 45 seconds
   - ☐ 30 seconds   ☐ 1 minute
5. I can do the back glide.
6. I can do the back float and kick my feet.

   I can move through the water for ____ feet.

10

Look at the pictures and check the correct box.

I Know What To Do In the Water!

Is this child ___ calm or ___ panicked?

Is this child ___ calm or ___ panicked?

Is this child ___ calm or ___ panicked?

Is this child ___ calm or ___ panicked?

Is this child ___ calm or ___ panicked?

Is this child ___ calm or ___ panicked?

11

Safety Considerations

- Arrange your drills so students do not glide into wall or into each other.
- Stay within a body length of all swimmers in your class.
- Never turn your back on students.
- Keep yourself between your students and deep water.
- Always enter feet first into shallow water. Set a good example!
- Know your Emergency Action Plan.

Adventure Objectives

movement through the water; changing directions; safety rules

Learning Objectives

- Swimmers will practice floating and kicking from previous lesson.
- Swimmers will move through the water in a face-down position.
- Swimmers will push off wall to teacher.
- Swimmers will push back to wall using arm and leg movements.
- Swimmers will fall/jump off side to teacher.
- Swimmers will fall/jump off side and return unassisted.
- Swimmers will lift their heads first vertically and then horizontally to take breaths.

Procedure

- Read *Seal's Rock*.
- Begin journey by falling off Seal's Rock, picking up animals from the bottom, and kicking back to the side.
- Introduce arm motion while standing on bottom.
- Have swimmers bend over and pull water to their bodies.
- Introduce sequence: hold breath, float, kick, pull.
- Have swimmers execute sequence for a distance of six feet.
- Have swimmers fall/jump from side to teacher.
- Have swimmers fall/jump in, lift head for breath and return to he side.
- Introduce sequence: hold breath, float, kick, pull, lift for breath.

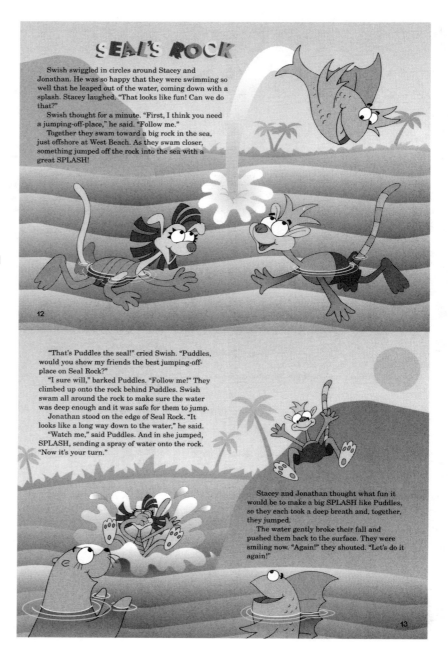

SEAL'S ROCK

Swish swiggled in circles around Stacey and Jonathan. He was so happy that they were swimming so well that he leaped out of the water, coming down with a splash. Stacey laughed. "That looks like fun! Can we do that?"

Swish thought for a minute. "First, I think you need a jumping-off-place," he said. "Follow me."

Together they swam toward a big rock in the sea, just offshore at West Beach. As they swam closer, something jumped off the rock into the sea with a great SPLASH!

"That's Puddles the seal!" cried Swish. "Puddles, would you show my friends the best jumping-off-place on Seal Rock?"

"I sure will," barked Puddles. "Follow me!" They climbed up onto the rock behind Puddles. Swish swam all around the rock to make sure the water was deep enough and it was safe for them to jump.

Jonathan stood on the edge of Seal Rock. "It looks like a long way down to the water," he said.

"Watch me," said Puddles. And in she jumped, SPLASH, sending a spray of water onto the rock. "Now it's your turn."

Stacey and Jonathan thought what fun it would be to make a big SPLASH like Puddles, so they each took a deep breath and, together, they jumped.

The water gently broke their fall and pushed them back to the surface. They were smiling now. "Again!" they shouted. "Let's do it again!"

Instructor Questions

1. Where do your feet need to go when you want to take a breath?
2. What did Swish and Puddles make sure of before jumping in the water?
3. How can your arms and legs help you move through the water?
4. What happens when you float on your stomach and steer with your arms?
5. After you jump in the water, how can you float on your back?
6. Where is the safest place to go after you jump in the water? How can you get there?

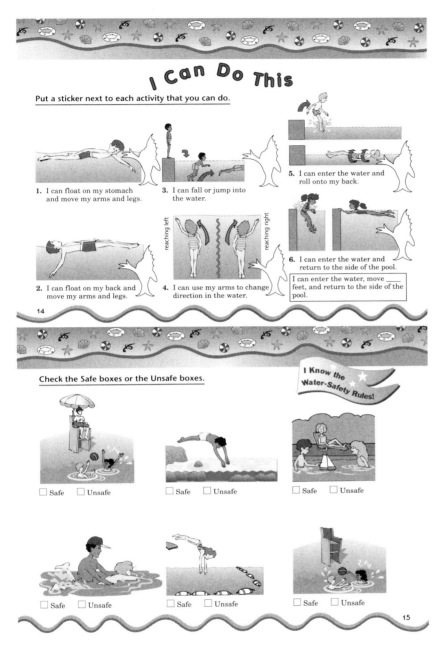

Teaching Tips

● Avoid holding students around the middle of the body in either front or back float. Assist by balancing at the head or shoulders.

● If the head is back with the ears in the water, "belly up, toes down" will help most students find the balance point for the backfloat.

● Walking backward while helping a student learn to float will create an eddy under their body that will help keep them afloat, as well as teach them movement.

Safety Considerations

● Gear all activities in this adventure to going back to the wall, rather than away.

● Stand next to the wall as students jump to make sure they jump out far enough.

● Stay within a body length of your group.

● Never turn your back on your students.

● Keep yourself between your students and deep water.

● Always enter feet first into shallow water. Set a good example!

● Know your Emergency Action Plan.

Adventure Objectives

coordinated stroke/crawl; ocean safety

Learning Objectives

- Swimmers will practice combined stroke on front and back.
- Swimmers will begin assisted breathing.
- Swimmers will improve crawl stroke, with arms recovering out of water.
- Swimmers will begin alternate breathing.
- Swimmers will swim a distance of twenty feet, using crawl stroke with alternate breathing.
- Swimmers will improve flutter kick mechanics.

Procedures

1. Read *Seaweed Patch*.
2. Review floating, kicking, and stroking on front and back.
3. Practice rotating from ear to face with even timing.
4. Have swimmers practice stroking and breathing while standing on the bottom.
5. Have swimmers practice front stroking, this time attempting to breathe. Offer support if necessary.
6. Have swimmers attempt to recover with one arm out of the water, then the other arm, then alternate arms, elbows high.
7. On a three count, introduce alternate breathing with out-of-water recovery.
8. Gradually increase distance using above skills.
9. When a swimmer can move a distance of twenty feet using the flutter kick, out-of-water recovery crawl, and alternate breathing, move to next adventure.

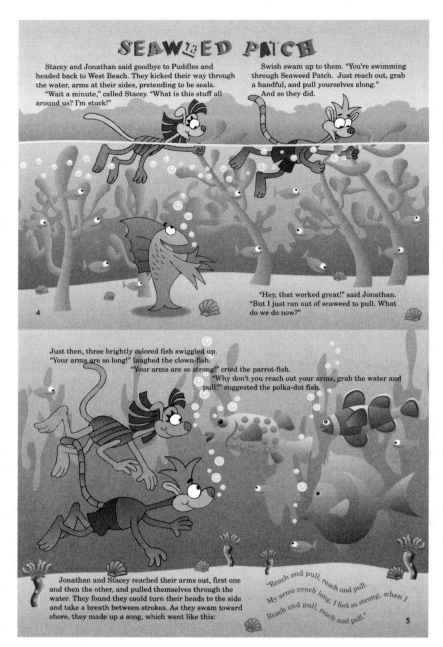

Instructor Questions

1. How can you get air when one of your ears is in the water?
2. When you roll your face into the water, if you breathe out, what happens?
3. What do your knees and toes do when you kick?
4. What happened when Stacey and Jonathan grabbed seaweed and pulled on it? What will happen if you grab some water and move it behind you?
5. Do your elbows stay bent when you pull water under you?
6. What part of your head is in the water when you breathe? What comes after your breath?

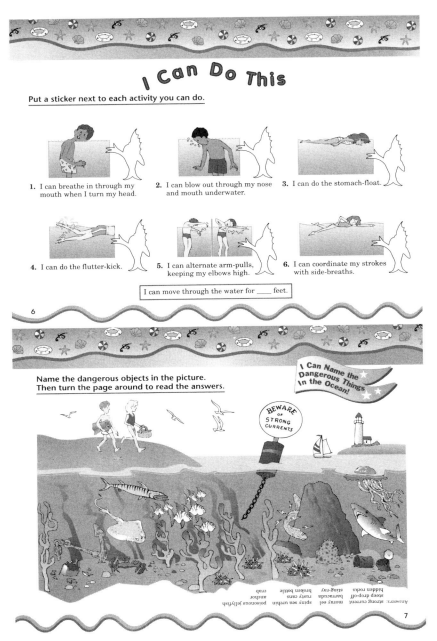

I Can Do This

Put a sticker next to each activity you can do.

1. I can breathe in through my mouth when I turn my head.

2. I can blow out through my nose and mouth underwater.

3. I can do the stomach-float.

4. I can do the flutter-kick.

5. I can alternate arm-pulls, keeping my elbows high.

6. I can coordinate my strokes with side-breaths.

I can move through the water for _____ feet.

6

Name the dangerous objects in the picture.
Then turn the page around to read the answers.

I Can Name the Dangerous Things In the Ocean!

BEWARE OF STRONG CURRENTS

Answers: strong current; steep drop-off; hidden rocks; broken bottle; sting-ray; barracuda; rusty cans; moray eel; anchor; spiny sea urchin; poisonous jellyfish; crab

7

Teaching Tips

- Kick should be from hip, toes pointed.
- Emphasize up phase of kick.
- Encourage small, fast kicks.
- Check for blowing air out under water.
- Emphasize body roll with breathing, not just turning head.
- Rolling all the way on the back to breathe is a good lead-up drill.
- Hand enters in front of shoulder, pull under center of body, thumb touches thigh on exit.
- Smooth and efficient. No splash entry.
- Fins are a good teaching aid for these skills.

Safety Considerations

- Stay within a body length of all swimmers in your class.
- If using fins, be sure students put them on at pool's edge, and do not walk on the deck with fins on.
- Never turn your back on your students.
- Keep yourself between your students and deep water.
- Always enter feet first into shallow water. Set a good example!
- Know your Emergency Action Plan.

Adventure Objectives

movement through water on back; boating safety

Learning objectives

- Swimmers will float on back in a relaxed manner.
- Swimmers will learn to stand from a back float.
- Swimmers will learn to kick while floating on their backs.
- Swimmers will use both legs and arms while in the back float position.
- Swimmers will push off on their backs, roll to their stomachs, and return to the side.
- Swimmers will roll from their stomachs to their backs.

Procedures

1. Read *Otter's Cove*.
2. Review breath holding and exhaling techniques.
3. Begin by falling backwards while standing in water.
4. Place arms over the head, hold breath, and arch backwards very gently.
5. Repeat procedure 4. until swimmers' faces remain out of water and floating is relaxed
6. After back float is accomplished, have swimmer begin kicking slowly, then harder.
7. While standing, have swimmers practice back arm stroke.
8. Introduce sequence: back float, add kick, then arms.
9. Have swimmers push off side, pick up animals from bottom, surface, float on back, place animals on their chests and swim to the side of the pool. When this is done five times, move on to the next adventure.

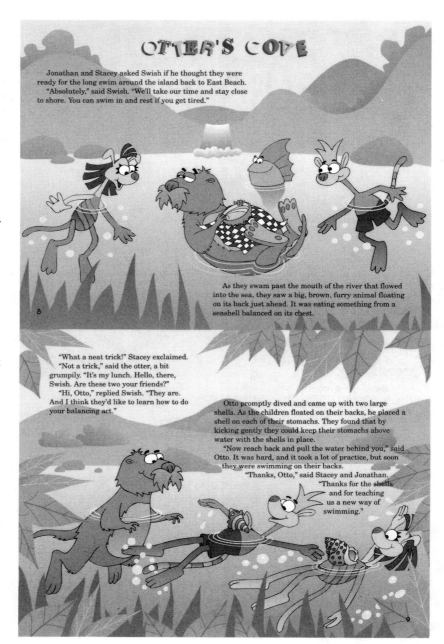

OTTER'S COVE

Jonathan and Stacey asked Swish if he thought they were ready for the long swim around the island back to East Beach. "Absolutely," said Swish. "We'll take our time and stay close to shore. You can swim in and rest if you get tired."

As they swam past the mouth of the river that flowed into the sea, they saw a big, brown, furry animal floating on its back just ahead. It was eating something from a seashell balanced on its chest.

"What a neat trick!" Stacey exclaimed. "Not a trick," said the otter, a bit grumpily. "It's my lunch. Hello, there, Swish. Are these two your friends?" "Hi, Otto," replied Swish. "They are. And I think they'd like to learn how to do your balancing act."

Otto promptly dived and came up with two large shells. As the children floated on their backs, he placed a shell on each of their stomachs. They found that by kicking gently they could keep their stomachs above water with the shells in place. "Now reach back and pull the water behind you," said Otto. It was hard, and it took a lot of practice, but soon they were swimming on their backs. "Thanks, Otto," said Stacey and Jonathan. "Thanks for the shells and for teaching us a new way of swimming."

Instructor Questions

1. How can Otto hold a shell on his stomach? What happens to the shell when he rolls over?
2. How can you kick your feet while floating on your back without losing your "shell"?
3. As you stroke your arms while floating on your back, when do you pull and when do you push?
4. What can your legs do to help you move?
5. Tell me about how your arms and legs move together.

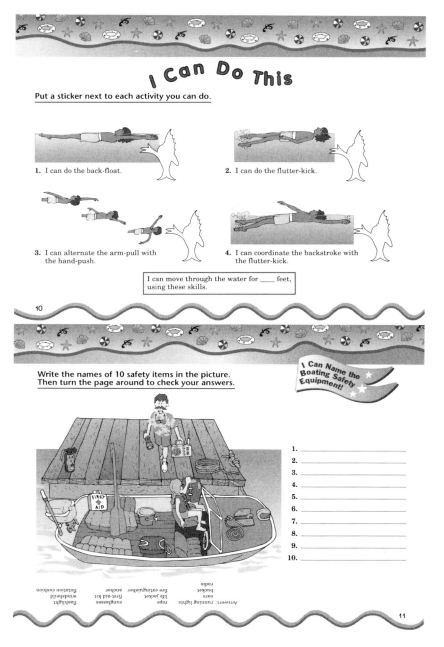

I Can Do This

Put a sticker next to each activity you can do.

1. I can do the back-float.
2. I can do the flutter-kick.
3. I can alternate the arm-pull with the hand-push.
4. I can coordinate the backstroke with the flutter-kick.

I can move through the water for ____ feet, using these skills.

10

Write the names of 10 safety items in the picture. Then turn the page around to check your answers.

I Can Name the Boating Safety Equipment!

1. _____
2. _____
3. _____
4. _____
5. _____
6. _____
7. _____
8. _____
9. _____
10. _____

Answers: running lights, radio, oars, bucket, fire extinguisher, anchor, rope, life jacket, first-aid kit, sunglasses, flotation cushion, windshield, flashlight

11

Teaching Tips

- Emphasize up kick, push water with top of foot.
- Small, fast kicks.
- Little finger enters first.
- Catch water, pull to waist, then push.
- Head still!
- Brush ear with arm as it enters.
- Fins are a helpful teaching aid.

Safety Considerations

- Arrange drills so swimmers do not swim backward into walls, or contact a swimmer coming in the opposite direction.
- Young learners will have difficulty swimming in a straight line.
- If using fins, be sure students put them on at pool's edge and do not walk on deck with fins on.
- Never turn your back on your students.
- Keep yourself between your students and deep water.
- Always enter feet first into shallow water. Set a good example!
- Know your Emergency Action Plan.

Adventure Objectives

coordinated stroking (breast stroke); home pool safety.

Learning Objectives

- Swimmers will hold onto side of pool and practice kick while on stomachs.
- Swimmers will practice arm movement while standing first, then leaning over and pulling water.
- Swimmers will review float on stomach.
- Swimmers will execute sequence: float, pull/breathe, kick and glide.
- Swimmers will repeat sequence for distance of ten feet.

Procedure

1. Read *Tadpole Pool*.
2. Have swimmers float on their stomach and practice kick while holding onto side of pool.
3. Practice kick only, while holding breath. (Note: to begin with, tadpoles only have legs.)
4. Practice arms while standing. ('Tadpoles' arms are very short.)
5. Introduce breathing as part of the arm motion.
6. Introduce sequence: float, pull and breathe, then kick and glide. (Note: arms and legs move at different times.)
7. When swimmers can move a distance of ten feet using this sequence, move to next adventure.

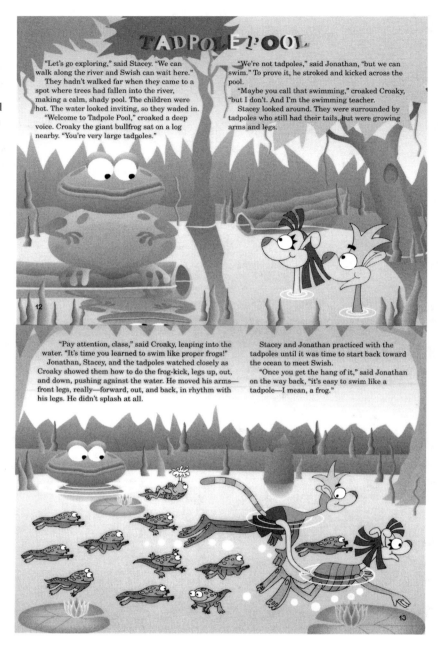

Instructor Questions

1. What do you think it looks like when a frog kicks?
2. How do tadpoles move if they don't have arms?
3. How do frogs move without splashing?
4. Tell me about your knees and your feet when you kick like a frog.
5. Tell me how you can pull and kick. What comes first? Next? Last?
6. How do you look when you start the stroke?
7. How do you look when you end the stroke?

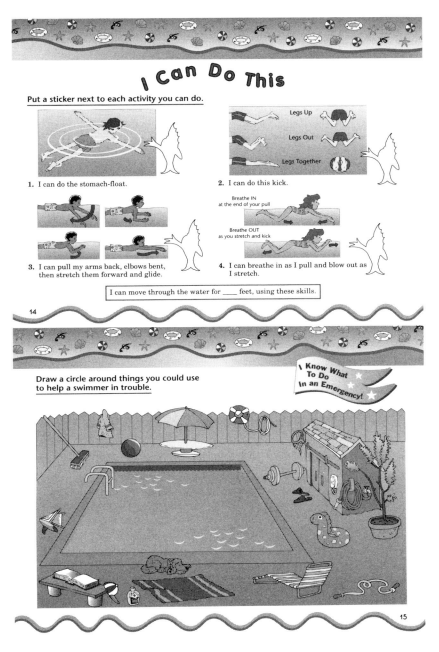

I Can Do This

Put a sticker next to each activity you can do.

1. I can do the stomach-float.

Legs Up
Legs Out
Legs Together

2. I can do this kick.

3. I can pull my arms back, elbows bent, then stretch them forward and glide.

Breathe IN
at the end of your pull

Breathe OUT
as you stretch and kick

4. I can breathe in as I pull and blow out as I stretch.

I can move through the water for ____ feet, using these skills.

14

Draw a circle around things you could use to help a swimmer in trouble.

I Know What To Do In an Emergency!

15

Teaching Tips

- Use kick, stretch, pull timing cues if swimmer is having difficulty with timing by starting with pull.
- Knees should not be wider than the hips.
- Lift heels to rear, toes out, push legs back to start.
- Elbows high.
- Trace or tape the pull pattern on a wall or bench to practice on land.
- Beginner drill: palms push to sides of pool, little finger up, touch chest, stretch out.
- Pull should not go past chest. Keep arms in front of body.

Safety Considerations

- Review how to recover from a front float/glide; back float glide.
- Review deep-water skills (treading, recovery).
- Organize drills and practice for maximum class control.
- Avoid letting your swimmers get to spread out if practicing/drilling over a long length of the pool.
- Never turn your back on your students.
- Keep yourself between your students and deep water.
- Always enter feet first into shallow water. Set a good example!
- Know your Emergency Action Plan.

Adventure Objectives

coordinated stroking (elementary back); water safety rules.

Learning Objectives

- Swimmers will practice both kick and arm motion for elementary back while sitting on the side.
- Swimmers will back float.
- Swimmers will practice elementary back kick while holding onto side.
- Swimmers will execute sequence: float, kick, then arms and glide.
- Swimmers will repeat sequence for a distance of ten feet.

Procedures

1. Read *Frog Pond.*
2. Have swimmers squat like frogs and jump.
3. Point out the similar leg positions in squat and elementary back kick, i.e., both legs move at the same time.
4. Have swimmers make a cross with arms.
5. Have swimmers stand up straight.
6. Introduce sequence squat/cross, then standing up straight.
7. Move to water and practice float.
8. Introduce sequence float, squat/cross then stand up straight. Note: keep buttocks up.
9. When swimmers can move a distance of ten feet, move on to next adventure.

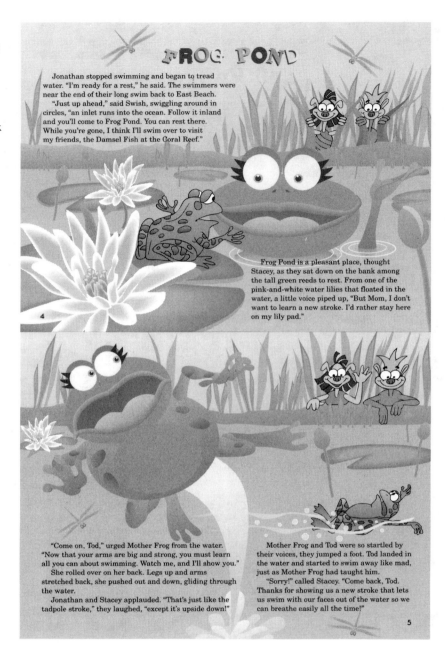

FROG POND

Jonathan stopped swimming and began to tread water. "I'm ready for a rest," he said. The swimmers were near the end of their long swim back to East Beach.

"Just up ahead," said Swish, swiggling around in circles, "an inlet runs into the ocean. Follow it inland and you'll come to Frog Pond. You can rest there. While you're gone, I think I'll swim over to visit my friends, the Damsel Fish at the Coral Reef."

4

Frog Pond is a pleasant place, thought Stacey, as they sat down on the bank among the tall green reeds to rest. From one of the pink-and-white water lilies that floated in the water, a little voice piped up, "But Mom, I don't want to learn a new stroke. I'd rather stay here on my lily pad."

"Come on, Tod," urged Mother Frog from the water. "Now that your arms are big and strong, you must learn all you can about swimming. Watch me, and I'll show you."

She rolled over on her back. Legs up and arms stretched back, she pushed out and down, gliding through the water.

Jonathan and Stacey applauded. "That's just like the tadpole stroke," they laughed, "except it's upside down!"

Mother Frog and Tod were so startled by their voices, they jumped a foot. Tod landed in the water and started to swim away like mad, just as Mother Frog had taught him.

"Sorry!" called Stacey. "Come back, Tod. Thanks for showing us a new stroke that lets us swim with our faces out of the water so we can breathe easily all the time!"

5

Instructor Questions

1. How can you rest and breathe at the same time like Jonathan and Stacey?
2. When Tod moved through the water on his back, what did his legs do?
3. When did his legs bend? Straighten?
4. Can you row your arms in the water? After a row, how far does your body glide?
5. When Tod did the elementary back stroke, what came first? Next? Last? How long did he glide?
6. How can you rest when you do this stroke? Is it easy to breathe?

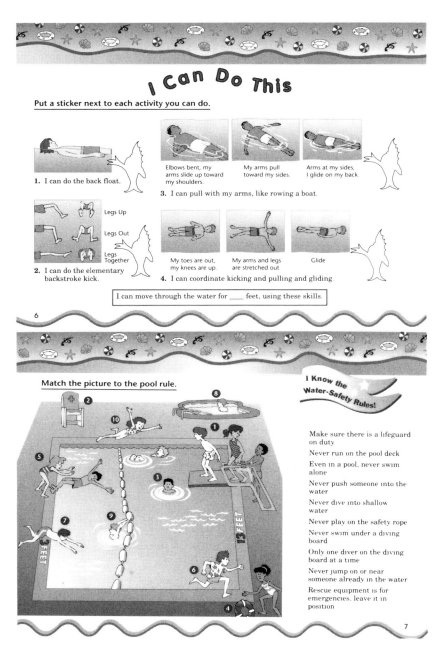

I Can Do This

Put a sticker next to each activity you can do.

1. I can do the back float.

Elbows bent, my arms slide up toward my shoulders.

My arms pull toward my sides.

Arms at my sides, I glide on my back.

3. I can pull with my arms, like rowing a boat.

Legs Up

Legs Out

Legs Together

2. I can do the elementary backstroke kick.

My toes are out, my knees are up.

My arms and legs are stretched out.

Glide

4. I can coordinate kicking and pulling and gliding.

I can move through the water for _____ feet, using these skills.

6

Match the picture to the pool rule.

I Know the Water-Safety Rules!

Make sure there is a lifeguard on duty

Never run on the pool deck

Even in a pool, never swim alone

Never push someone into the water

Never dive into shallow water

Never play on the safety rope

Never swim under a diving board

Only one diver on the diving board at a time

Never jump on or near someone already in the water

Rescue equipment is for emergencies, leave it in position

7

Teaching Tips

- Fingertips slide up body to armpits, then out and pull. (As if zippers run up the side of the body.)
- Beginners will want to move arms continuously—emphasize holding thighs after pulling to force glide.
- Thighs stay near the surface on kick, bottom half of leg drops down, toes out, squeeze legs back together.
- Knees stay underwater.

Teaching Tips

- Fingertips slide up body to armpits, then out and pull. (As if zippers run up the side of the body.)
- Beginners will want to move arms continuously—emphasize holding thighs after pulling to force glide.
- Thighs stay near the surface on kick, bottom half of leg drops down, toes out, squeeze legs back together.
- Knees stay underwater.

Safety Considerations

- Young learners will have difficulty swimming in a straight line.
- Arrange your drills so students do not glide into wall or each other.
- Review how to recover from a front float/glide; back float glide.
- Review deep-water skills (treading, recovery).
- Organize drills and practice for maximum class control.
- Never turn your back on your students.
- Keep yourself between your students and deep water.
- Always enter feet first into shallow water. Set a good example!
- Know your Emergency Action Plan.

Adventure Objectives

coordinated stroking (butterfly); water safety decision making.

Learning Objectives

- Swimmers will improve crawl stroke with alternate breathing.
- Swimmers will learn two-handed crawl, with head up.
- Swimmers will learn two-handed crawl, with breathing on alternate sides.
- Swimmers will learn dolphin kick.
- Swimmers will practice dolphin kick with bobbing for breath.
- Swimmers will swim a distance of ten feet using two-handed crawl, dolphin kick, and bob breathing.

Procedures

1. Read *Dolphin's Den*.
2. Review crawl stroke with alternate breathing.
3. Have swimmers move both arms together while swimming crawl.
4. Have swimmers practice two-handed crawl, head up, head down, breathing to the side.
5. Have swimmers practice flutter kick with both legs together.
6. Work kick only, arms to the side, and bob for breath.
7. Teach sequence: dolphin kick, two-handed crawl, bob for breath.
8. When swimmers can move a distance of ten feet using the sequence, move to next adventure.

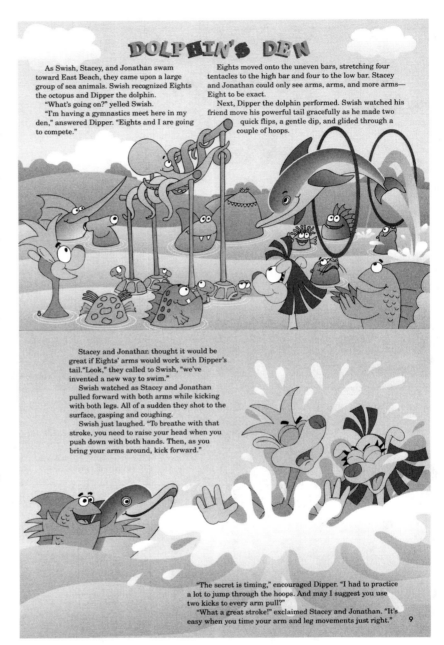

Instructor Questions

1. What happens if you do the crawl arm stroke with both arms at the same time? Do your arms stay wet all the time?
2. When you dolphin kick, what do your legs do when your arms go in the water? What do your legs do when your hands get under your chest?
3. How many kicks did Dipper say to do with each arm stroke? What do the kicks help you to do?
4. What part of your body starts the downward movement of your body?

78

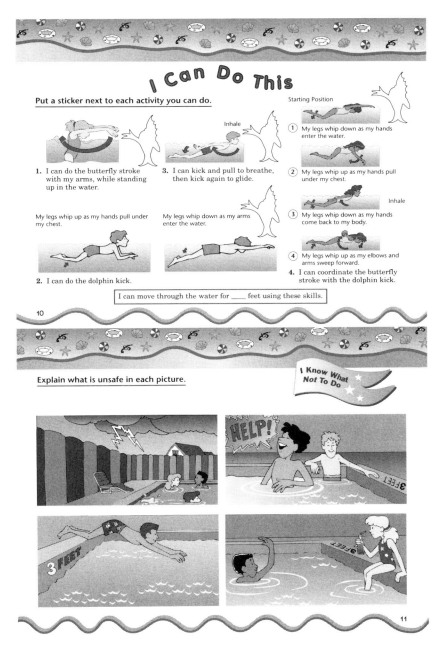

- Dolphin kick drills on the back help develop the feel of the kick.
- The head leads the downward movement.
- Wall drill: stand five feet from the pool wall with legs and feet together. Bump rear against wall, then push stomach forward.
- Dolphin dives pushing off bottom.
- Key phrase: head before hands.
- Butterfly stroke should not be portrayed as being more difficult than other strokes.
- Fins are a helpful teaching aid.

Safety Considerations

- Review treading water and deep-water safety skills before practicing in deep water.
- Arrange class flow and drills in single file to accommodate for the wide stroke recovery of the butterfly.
- If using fins, be sure students put them on at pool's edge and do not walk on the deck with fins on.
- Never turn your back on your students.
- Keep yourself between your students and deep water.
- Always enter feet first into shallow water. Set a good example!
- Know your Emergency Action Plan.

Adventure Objectives

coordinated stroking (side stroke); water safety decision making.

Learning Objectives

- Swimmers will rotate to side and convert side flutter kick to side scissor kick.
- Swimmers will move in water on side using arms.
- Swimmers will practice each arm motion independent of other arm.
- Swimmers will put arms and legs together.

Procedure

1. Tell *Flounder Farm* story.
2. Using a kickboard or other aid, practice kicking on the side.
3. Once movement is achieved, modify the kick to a scissor kick.
4. Holding onto the kickboard, practice each arm movement individually.
5. Holding onto the kickboard, practice the scissor kick and top arm motion.
6. Now reverse and hold the kickboard with the top arm, then kick and pull with the bottom arm.
7. Once the individual motions are learned, teach the sequence: stroke, kick, and glide.

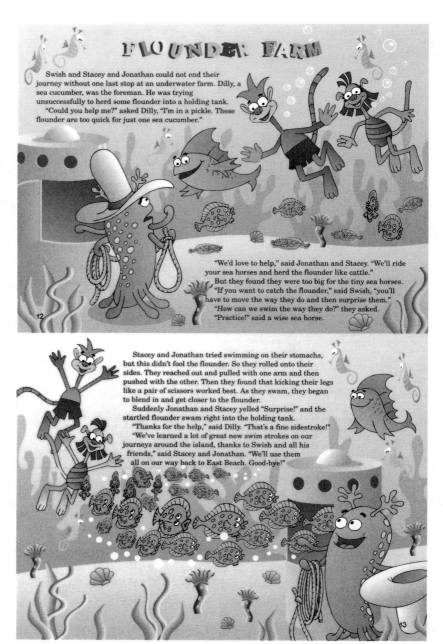

Instructor Questions

1. How is a flounder different from other fish?
2. What ways can you move through the water like a flounder?
3. When you do sidestroke, tell me about your arms and legs. When do you glide?
4. When you scissor your legs, in which direction does your top leg go? Does it matter if it goes forward or backward?
5. How about your arms? Do they pull at the same time? Which arm is stretched above your head?

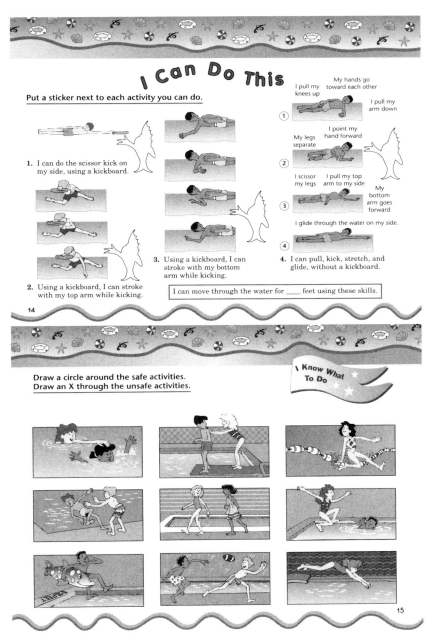

I Can Do This

Put a sticker next to each activity you can do.

1. I can do the scissor kick on my side, using a kickboard.

2. Using a kickboard, I can stroke with my top arm while kicking.

3. Using a kickboard, I can stroke with my bottom arm while kicking.

4. I can pull, kick, stretch, and glide, without a kickboard.

(1) I pull my knees up — My hands go toward each other — I pull my arm down

(2) My legs separate — I point my hand forward

(3) I scissor my legs — I pull my top arm to my side — My bottom arm goes forward

(4) I glide through the water on my side.

I can move through the water for ____ feet using these skills.

14

Teaching Tips

- Slow, easy movements.
- No splash.
- Emphasize glide.
- Push top shoulder back to get on side.

Draw a circle around the safe activities.
Draw an X through the unsafe activities.

I Know What To Do

15

Safety Considerations

- Review proper use of kickboard.
- Avoid letting your swimmers get too spread out if practicing/drilling over a long length of the pool.
- Review treading water and deep-water safety skills if practicing in deep water for the first time.
- Never turn your back on your students.
- Keep yourself between your students and deep water.
- Always enter feet first into shallow water. Set a good example!
- Know your Emergency Action Plan.

Part 3
Challenge Program

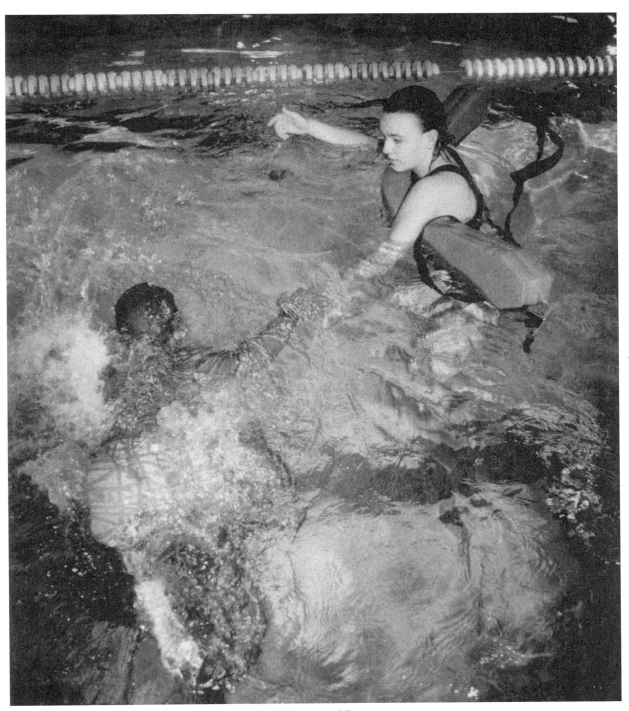

PROGRAM OVERVIEW

The Challenge component of the Learn to Swim program encompasses the full range of aquatic skills appropriate for life-long enjoyment of the water. There are three parts to the program, the Stroke & Safety Challenge, Fitness Challenge, and Sprint Challenge. The program is administered on the local level, by a Program Coordinator, who is responsible for quality control, for the safety of participants, and for training instructors. Instructors conduct the swimming classes under the guidance of the program coordinator, maintaining a ratio of students per instructor that allows for safety and an appropriate environment for students to meet performance objectives. Instructors teach the Stroke & Safety class with the objective to analyze performance and assist the student in progressing toward skilled movement. Performance for each skill is evaluated at three levels-novice, advanced, and expert. The "challenge" to the student is to work toward achieving a higher performance level. Charts and award certificates help monitor performance level and progress through the skills. The Fitness Challenge offers instructors creative methods of introducing students to life-long participation in swimming to improve conditioning level. The Swim The Seven Seas program offers participants a means to tracking distance, with an awards system designed to keep motivation high. The Sprint Challenge offers participants an introduction into competitive swimming, while also improving skill development through speed work.

PROGRAM COORDINATORS
Program coordinators are trained and licensed by Jeff Ellis & Associates, Inc. Coordinators will be held accountable for maintaining the established standard of care and programs will be randomly and independently audited by Jeff Ellis & Associates to ensure compliance. Coordinators conduct instructor training according to their facility needs.

INSTRUCTORS
Instructors may train for, and be certified to teach any or all of the Challenge components. Time involvement for instructor training is dependent upon the experience of the instructor and is at the discretion of the Program Coordinator. All instructor training must be documented and kept on file for as long as the Learn to Swim program is offered.

STUDENTS
Students in the Learn to Swim Challenge program may be of any age appropriate for the activities being offered. Generally, students will be ages 8 - adult. The program may be customized to encompass any age group, performance level, and course structure, depending upon the needs of the facility.

INTRODUCTION

Safety is the primary concern of the challenge series. Certainly , water poses an obvious hazard in which to learn any activity. The rules that follow are common sense tips for any activity around the water.

1. **Never swim alone. Always conduct aquatic activities in pairs or in a supervised area.**
2. **Know your personal limits when it comes to aquatic activities. Don't over estimate your abilities in the water.**
3. **Familiarize yourself with the aquatic environment before you enter the water.**
4. **Always pay attention to warning signs or instructions that are present at an aquatic sight.**

The above rules seem very simple, however in their broadest context they are the areas, when neglected, that lead to most injuries or fatalities in aquatics. There is no complete source of specific rules or regulations that covers all aquatic situations. Better yet the general objective of _safety in the aquatic environment_ is much more desirable than trying to anticipate specific unsafe situations in or around an aquatic facility.

In addition to obvious traditional safety concerns, also be aware of personal precautions that should be taken in preparation and execution of all aquatic skills.

1. **Always "warm-up" before any type of physical activity. Failure to properly warm-up may result in injury. This is a consideration with swimmers of all ages.**
2. **Always try to execute the skill in the proper manner as described by the instructor. Improper skill execution can lead to injury.**
3. **Monitor fatigue. Although a combination of other concerns mentioned, fatigue is always an enemy of any athlete. Failure to recognize excess fatigue can lead to injury and possible fatality.**
4. **Adopt a reasonable "Learning/Training " progression. While pushing ones self to the limit, on occasion, is desirable, a progression that is excessive to the individual leads to a point of diminishing returns. In addition, fatigue and improper skill execution will usually result.**

Once again these rules seem very simple, however if not adhered to much long-term injury can result. Things to consider before you start:

1. What physical shape are you in?
2. Why are you doing this? recreation-safety-skill improvement-exercise
3. What do you expect out of the program?
4. What kind of time can you give to the program?

Stroke & Safety Component

BODY POSITIONS PERFORMANCE EVALUATION

FLOATING:

Floating is the basis of all body positions for swimming. Swimmers must be able to float on the front, back and both sides. In addition, floating is the key to personal safety in the water. Having learned the level of comfort that can be achieved with a float, many swimmers can avoid the overexertion and fatigue that often results in aquatic emergencies.

GLIDING:

Gliding is the basis for streamlining, and streamlining is the basis for momentum in all swimming strokes. A relaxed glide on the stomach, back and side is the key to maximum forward momentum with minimum effort.

Front float performed at the novice level

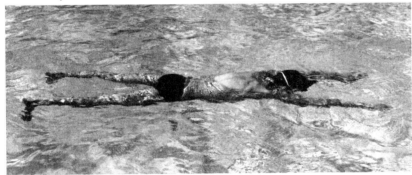

Front float performed at the expert level

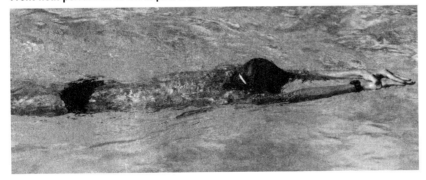

SKILLS
FRONT FLOAT:

1. Take a breath and hold it.
2. Put your face in the water.
3. Allow your body to relax.
4. Arms extended to the side
5. Lie flat on the water.
6. Raise feet off the bottom.
7. Maintain position for a brief count.

NOVICE:
1. Body might not be horizontal.
2. Arms may be bent.
3. Legs may not be horizontal.
4. Float maintained for short period of time.

ADVANCED:
1. Body must be nearly horizontal.
2. Arms must be almost straight.
3. Legs must be nearly horizontal.
4. Float maintained for an extended period of time.

EXPERT:
1. Body must be horizontal.
2. Arms must be fully extended.
3. Legs are horizontal.
4. Except for breathing, float maintained indefinitely.

87

BACK FLOAT:

1. Take a breath and hold it.
2. Allow your body to relax.
3. Extend your arms to the sides slightly higher than the shoulders.
4. Arch your back and lie on the water.
5. Legs should be raised, relaxed and extended.
6. Face should be out of the water, chin up, head back.
7. Maintain position for a brief count.

SIDE FLOAT:
(Bottom Photo)

1. Take a breath and hold it.
2. Allow your body to relax.
3. Extend one arm over your head, the other along your side.
4. Gently lean to side of the arm over the head and lie on the water.
5. Legs should be raised, relaxed and extended.

TEACHING TIPS:

1. Chest deep water works best when learning floats. Shallow water tends to lead to " jumping on top of the water" thus sinking.
2. Aids such as the side of pool, floats, and instructors supporting students may be needed.

DRILL:

1. Begin each class with swimmers floating in all three positions. While floating, slowly lift the head, then an arm, then a leg. See what effect these actions have on the float.

Back float performed at the novice level.

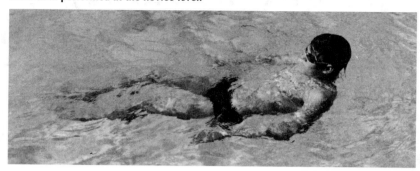

Back float performed at the advanced level.

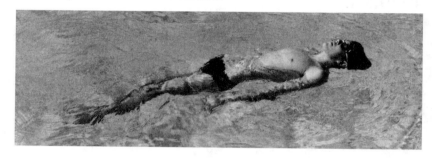

Back float performed at the expert level.

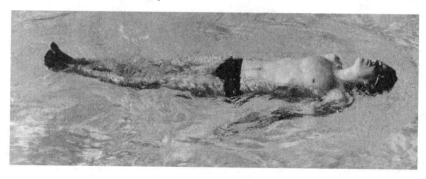

Side float is an important lead-up to freestyle breathing.

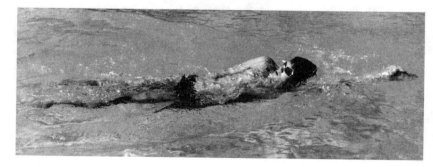

FREESTYLE/CRAWL STROKE

The crawl stroke is both the fastest and most efficient of the swimming strokes. The ability to perform the crawl is useful in recreation, competitive swimming, and personal safety.

Allow for body roll during the entire stroke.

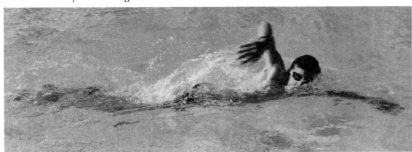

High elbow recovery, hand entering in line with the shoulder, good catch of the water and a center line pull are elements of freestyle at the expert level.

TIPS:
1. Water should cut the body in half.
2. Legs should be straight but not ridged, ankles should be loose.
3. Elbow should be bent during pull and recovery.
4. Inhale at the end of the pull, exhale through the nose and mouth.
5. Allow for some body roll during entire stroke.

Inhale at the end of the pull.

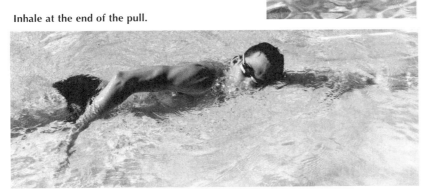

DRILLS:
1. Practice kick with a kick board fully extended.
2. Using board pull with one arm, using 6 beat kick.
3. Swim with thumbs under armpit to achieve bent elbow.

BODY POSITION:
1. The swimmer is in a front float.
2. The water surface cuts the body in half.
Note: This will vary depending on body composition.

LEGS:
1. Kick alternately up and down.
2. Kick originates from the hip.
3. Kick is a fluid action of the lower leg, ankle and foot.
4. The toes are pointed backward.

ARMS:
1. Arms alternate.
2. Bring one arm forward into water with elbow high.
3. Bend elbow as pull begins.
4. Pull in a center line underneath the body.
5. Lift arm out of water, elbow first.
6. Recover out of water, and bring arm forward.

BREATHING:
1. Inhale on breathing side as that arm is pulled back.
2. Exhale as arm is extended forward during first of pull.
Note: Alternate breathing (breathing on both sides) may even body movement.

COORDINATION:
1. Roughly, 6 kicks per arm cycle is desirable.

Note: This standard will vary according to individual body composition and preference.

2. Coordination should result in efficient forward motion that is smooth and consistent.

NOVICE:
1. Body might not be horizontal.
2. Kick may not be continuous, may pump or be to the side.
3. Arms sometimes recover under water, may pull wide, may be straight.
4. Breathing needs to be to the side, body rolling is permitted.
5. Must be comfortable in the water, poor coordination permitted.

ADVANCED:
1. Body near horizontal.
2. Kick continuous and at the surface most of the time.
3. Arms recover out of the water, pull close to center, occasionally straight.
4. Exhale under water, occasional rolling permitted.
5. Strong kick, arms coordinated with breathing, confident.

EXPERT:
1. Body must be horizontal.
2. Kick is continuous and all of the time.
3. Arms recover smooth, pull in center of body, elbow bent 90 degrees. Head rotates as little as possible for breath, body roll not permitted.
4. Strong kick at the surface, well coordinated smooth, efficient stroke.

FREESTYLE/CRAWL STROKE BREATHING

The key to this drill is keeping the number of strokes in between side glides very low, and consistent. A very effective drill sequence for teaching breathing that has been developed in Canada uses a "One-Two-Three-Breathe" pattern exclusively with excellent success. This pattern also teaches bi-lateral breathing, as the odd stroke count will put the body on alternating sides after each side-glide.

Side-Glide Breathing Drills

1. Practice side floats, on both sides of the body. The upper arm should be extended, with the students head touching the extended arm, and the chin pointed to the opposite shoulder. The mouth will be out of the water.
2. Add a freestyle/flutter kick to the side float.
3. Add the arm stroke by having the student reach forward with the top arm, and roll the body into a horizontal position. Complete 1, 2, or 3 strokes only.
4. When the hand enters the water on the designated stroke number, keep that arm extended, and roll the body back into the side glide position for a breath. Allow the student to stay in the side glide long enough to get enough breaths, and then continue the drill.
5. Shorten the length of time the student stays in the side-glide position to breathe.

Practice side-glide on both left and right sides. (Demonstrated in the top and middle photo.)

After the breath, begin the stroke by reaching forward with the top arm. (Shown in the bottom photo at right.)

Freestyle/Crawl stroke breathing can be easily taught by emphasizing the side glide position, and starting with the breath first...rather than emphasizing getting a breath after the pull. Begin introducing this side position to the student as soon as possible when teaching the freestyle/crawl stroke. Too often, instructors will try to teach side breathing by having a student keep the body horizontal and stationary (such as holding on to a wall or kickboard) while simply turning the head to breathe. This positioning makes the skill difficult to perform for the student, and does little to simulate what actually happens when swimming freestyle and integrating breathing into the stroke. Properly performed, breathing will occur as the shoulders and upper torso rotate into a side glide position.

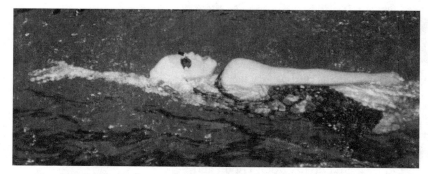

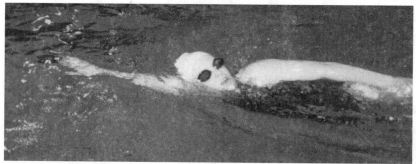

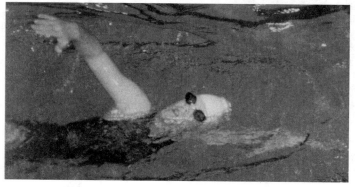

90

The backstroke is the third fastest stroke. It is the only stroke where the face never truly enters the water. As a result breathing is much easier, and for some, it is an easier stroke to learn.

A streamlined body position is necessary for good backstroke, and makes an excellent kicking drill.

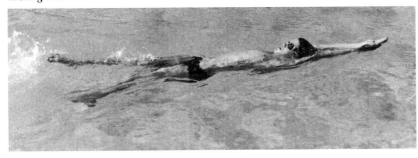

Arms should be in opposition to each other and allow for some body roll.

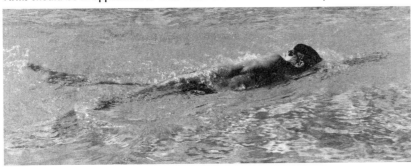

Arms should be straight on recovery, with the head back and still. Hand enters little finger first, parallel to midline of body.

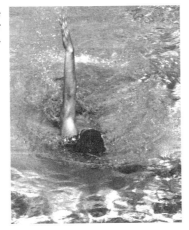

BODY POSITION:
1. The swimmer is in a back float.
2. Hips sink slightly below the surface of the water.
3. Head should be comfortably back.

LEGS:
1. Kick alternately up and down.
2. Leg is straight on the down kick.
3. Leg is bent on the up kick.
4. Only the toes should break the surface of the water.

ARMS:
1. Arms alternate.
2. Bring one arm out of the water, little finger first.
3. Hand enters the water. parallel to the body mid-line.
4. Press the hand outward and toward the feet.
5. Bend the elbow 90 degrees to allow the forearm to push
6. Recover out of the water.

BREATHING:
Even though the head is out of the water, a breathing pattern should be established. Inhaling during one arm stroke and exhaling on the other arm stroke is a common practice.

COORDINATION:
1. Arms should be in opposition to each other.
2. A 6 beat kick cycle is desirable.

NOVICE:
1. Head may be occasionally up, hips occasionally down.
2. Kick may pump, may not be continuous.
3. Arms may occasionally pull to the side.
4. No established pattern on breathing.
5. Must remain on back, poor coordination permitted.

ADVANCED:
1. Head and hips close to horizontal.
2. Kick continuous may occasionally break surface.
3. Arms reach straight to top of stroke, elbow bends during pull.
4. Begin breath pattern, may not be continuous.
5. Strong kick arms remain in opposition.

EXPERT:
1. Head and hips remain in horizontal position.
2. Kick strong and continuous, only toes break surface.
3. Arms reach to top of stroke consistently, elbow bend 90 degrees during pull.
4. Breath patten established and continuous.
5. Stroke well coordinated smooth and efficient.

TIPS:

1. Head should remain back during the stroke.
2. Legs should not break the surface during the kick.
3. Arms should be equal distance from body mid-line during reach.
4. Elbow should be at 90 degree angle during pull.
5. Allow for some body roll during stroke.

The backstroke is the third fastest stroke. It is the only stroke where the face never truly enters the water. As a result breathing is much easier, and for some, this makes it an easier stroke to learn.

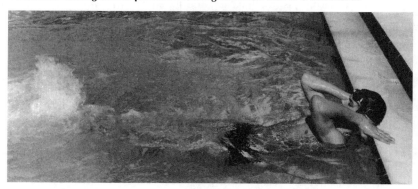

DRILLS:

1. Practice flutter kick while holding on to the side of the pool.
2. Practice flutter kick while holding on to a kick board.
3. Drill "S" pull while standing on the bottom.
4. Practice straight arm recovery.

ELEMENTARY BACKSTROKE

The elementary backstroke has implications both for personal safety and lifesaving techniques. Because you are on your back, there are no special breathing methods. Also, the arms and legs move at the same time which results in a glide or resting stage in this stroke.

Recover arms and legs at the same time

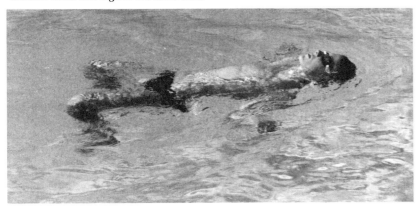

TIPS:
1. Keep the head back and hips up.
2. Recover the arms and legs at the same time.
3. Remain horizontal during the glide.

DRILLS:
1. Practice the kick only with a floatation device.
2. Practice arms only, keep legs straight.

BODY POSITION:
1. The swimmer is in a front float.
2. The head is tilted slightly forward.
3. The body should remain horizontal.

LEGS:
1. Bend knees and draw heels toward buttocks.
2. Turn feet out and circle them as you extend.
3. Legs should come together and toes are pointed.

ARMS:
1. Both arms recover at the same time.
2. Bend elbows and slide hands along body towards shoulders.
3. Once they reach the shoulders, extend the hands straight out like a cross.
4. Pull both hands towards the body keep the arms straight.

BREATHING:
While the face is out of the water during this stroke an established pattern of breathing will make it more efficient.

COORDINATION:
1. Begin with legs straight and arms by the side.
2. Draw knees toward the hips as you slide the hands toward the shoulders.
3. Turn feet out and extend legs out and around as arms extend and pull toward body.
4. A glide should result.

NOVICE:
1. Hips may drop, body not horizontal.
2. Legs may not recover together.
3. Arms may recover before or beyond shoulders.
4. Arms and legs may not move together.

ADVANCED:
1. Body mostly horizontal.
2. Scissor kick not acceptable.
3. Hands do not recover beyond head.
4. Arms and legs finish together.

EXPERT:
1. Body horizontal, hips and shoulders remain level.
2. Legs recover simultaneously, knees do not break surface.
3. Arms must be symmetrical and simultaneous throughout stroke.
4. Glide required, arms and legs finish together.

BREASTSTROKE

The breaststroke is the slowest of the competitive swimming strokes. However, this stroke is often learned by some much easier that the other strokes and its recreational value and safety value are important assets in learning the stroke correctly.

As the pull reaches the shoulders, bring the elbows together and extend the arms.

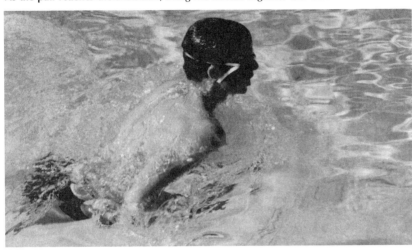

Inhaling occurs during the pull of the arms.

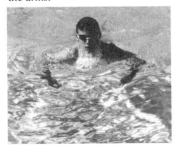

Legs should bend as the arms extend.

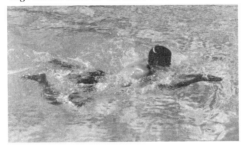

TIPS:
1. Elbows should be up for the pull.
2. Pull down as well as back.
3. Bend legs at hips and at knees.
4. Push feet out and back at the same time

DRILLS:
1. Practice kick only without a floatation device.
2. Practice 3 kicks to 1 pull.
3. Practice arms only with aid between legs.
4. To practice glide, count strokes then reduce the number.

BODY POSITION:
1. The swimmer is in a front float.
2. During execution of the stroke, the body will move up and down.
3. The head may submerge during the stroke.

LEGS:
1. Kick together, up, out and around.
2. Legs are bent so that feet come towards body.
3. Rotate feet outwards. kick out and back.
4. Bring feet together and point toes.

ARMS:
1. Arms pull together, down, out and back.
2. Hands pull to the side, down and back.
3. Bend elbows as the pull moves back.
4. As pull reaches the shoulders, bring the elbows together and extend the arms.

BREATHING:
1. Inhaling occurs during the pull of the arms.
2. Exhaling occurs during the extension of the arms.

COORDINATION:
1. Arms should pull as the legs extend.
2. Legs should bend as the arms extend.
3. Sequence is pull, kick and glide.

NOVICE:
1. Body may tilt during stroke.
2. Kick may not always be together.
3. Arms pull to side occasionally.
4. No established breathing pattern.
5. Must attempt paired action.

ADVANCED:
1. Body should remain level during most of the stroke.
2. Kick must be together, may not be streamlined.
3. Arm action must be paired, elbows bent.
4. Breath taken each stroke.
5. Kick and pull alternate.

EXPERT:
1. Body must be streamlined during glide.
2. Feet turn during kick and toes straight during glide.
3. Arms no wider than shoulder on pull, and not past shoulders.
4. Mouth on surface to inhale, exhale during arm extension.
5. Must have strong coordinated propulsion.

The butterfly is the last of the competitive strokes to be developed. This stroke uses a double overarm pull with a special kick called the dolphin kick. Both the arms and the legs execute their motion together. Upper body strength is an important part of this stroke.

The body will undulate during the stroke.

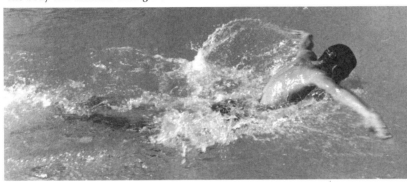

Inhaling occurs with the hands back and legs pushing down.

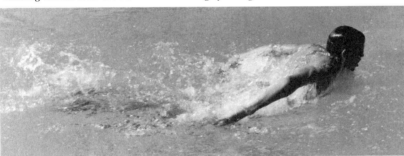

Don't lift too high to breath.

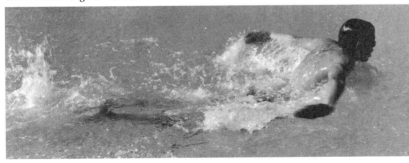

BODY POSITION:

1. The swimmer is in a front float.
2. Head is looking at the bottom of the pool.
3. The body will undulate during the stroke.

LEGS:

1. Kick together up and down.
2. Kick from the hips, knees flex and extend with kick.
3. Kick extension helps lift body for breath.
4. Toes are pointed during kick.

ARMS:

1. Arms move forward in an over hand motion.
2. Arms are pressed down and out with elbows high.
3. Hands continue around and press toward the hips.
4. Arms are swung over the surface on recovery.

BREATHING:

1. Inhaling occurs with hands back and legs pushing down
2. Exhaling occurs as hands pull under chest and legs move up.

COORDINATION:

1. As arms come out of the water, extend back forward, bend legs they should sink.
2. Pull arms down, straighten the legs.
3. Hands should reach hips as legs extend.
4. Two kicks to one stroke, one to reach, one to pull.

NOVICE:
1. Body may not be horizontal.
2. May have some flutter kicks.
3. Arms may not be together.
4. May hold stroke to breath.
5. Must attempt paired arm and leg action.

ADVANCED:
1. Body should be near horizontal.
2. Legs stay together.
3. Arms enter together, push to waist.
4. Exhale should be under water.
5. Must attempt 2 kicks to 1 pull.

EXPERT:
1. Body is horizontal.
2. Each stroke cycle has 2 strong kicks.
3. Arms should not pause during stroke.
4. Breath come at the end of the pull.
5. Continuous efficient stroke.

TIPS:
1. Keep legs together.
2. Bend elbows during pull.
3. Undulate body through stroke.
4. Don't lift too high to breath.

DRILLS:
1. Practice arms out of water or in front of a mirror
2. Practice dolphin kick on side or back.
3. Practice one arm only with dolphin kick.
4. Drill right arm left arm both arms with kick.

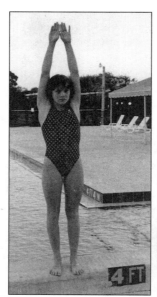

Practice the arm pull pattern out of water.

Arms in starting position.

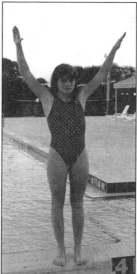

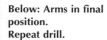

Arms in downward pulling position.

Below: Arms in final position.
Repeat drill.

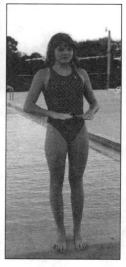

The side stroke like the elementary backstroke has a great deal of value as a relaxing stroke. Because the head remains out of the water, breathing is not an issue and the mixture of arm and leg movements makes a good distance stroke.

The mixture of arm and leg movements makes sidestroke a good distance stroke.

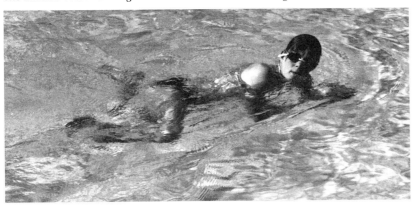

TIPS:
1. Keep head in line with body.
2. Arm and leg movements occur at the same time.
3. Emphasize the glide.

DRILLS:
1. Practice legs only on the side of the pool or with a kick board.
2. Practice both arm motions separately with a kick board.
3. Roll from one side to another and reach with the bottom arm.

BODY POSITION:
1. Body is horizontal on one side.
2. The arm nearest the pool bottom is extended over the head. The top arm rests at the side of the body.
3. Legs are together and extended.

LEGS:
1. Knees and legs are drawn toward hips.
2. Just below hips separate legs, one forward one back.
3. Scissor legs together and glide.

ARMS:
1. Bottom arm pulls down, top arm reaches forward.
2. Hands move toward each other.
3. Bottom arm moves forward, top arm pulls to side.

BREATHING:
The head remains out of the water during the stroke thus breathing is not an issue.

COORDINATION:
1. Start the stroke in the glide position.
2. As the move toward each other, the knees bend toward the hips.
3. The legs separate and the hands begin to pull apart.
4. As the legs scissor together the bottom arm moves forward and the top arm pull in front of the body.
5. The final part of the stroke is a glide on the side.

NOVICE:
1. Body may roll from side position,
2. Legs may not kick in the same place each time.
3. Arms may both reach forward and back at the same time.
4. Arms and leg may alternate.

ADVANCED:
1. Body should remain horizontal and on side.
2. Legs must be straight and together during glide.
3. Top arm and hand remain under water at all times.
4. Arms and legs must recover together.

EXPERT:
1. Head must remain in line with body.
2. Both legs remain horizontal during movements.
3. Pull with top arm is close to body, pull with lower arm is in line with body.
4. Extension of bottom arm results in glide which is streamlined.

TURNS

Whether the involvement in swimming is recreational or competitive there will no doubt come a time when an efficient turn will benefit that endeavor. Because there is a different objective for each, recreational and competitive turns are great deal of different.

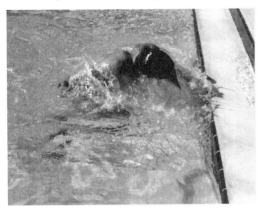

The objective of a good turn is to smoothly and effectively change direction.

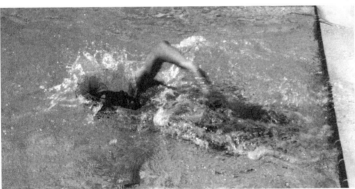

FRONT/SIDE
OPEN TURN:
This turn can be used with the front crawl or the side stroke.
1. Leading hand grabs the edge of the pool.
2. The feet are brought to the pool side, under the swimmer.
3. The body rotates and pushes away from the side.
4. The extension may be on the stomach or side depending on the stroke.

BACK OPEN TURN:
This turn may be used with either the back crawl or elementary backstroke.
1. Contact with the side of the pool is made with one arm extended.
2. As the legs are drawn toward the body, the head may submerge as the body rotates.
3. Legs make contact with the wall and push off as the arms are extended over the head.

RECREATIONAL
BREASTSTROKE Turn:
1. Although not essential, it is recommended that both hands touch the wall at the same time during this turn. This helps to maintain body position.
2. As contact is made with the side of the pool, the legs are brought under the body. Rotation of the body occurs and the legs push off with both arms extended.

101

COMPETITIVE TURNS

The nature of competitive turns is speed. For this reason, the body spends more time submerged than in open turns. There is less resistance under the surface of the water than at the surface.

CRAWL:

1. As you approach the wall tuck your head to begin a somersault.
2. As you pike through the somersault, tuck your legs as they reach the wall.
3. Push off the wall and rotate to your stomach.

BACKSTROKE:

1. As you approach the wall rotate to your stomach.
2. Tuck your head and begin a pike somersault.
3. Somersault to your back and push off with arms extended.

BUTTERFLY AND BREASTSTROKE:

1. Touch the wall with both arms fully extended and at the same time.
2. Tuck legs under the body and release the side of the pool as the feet contact the pool.
3. Rotate to your stomach and push off the side arms extended.

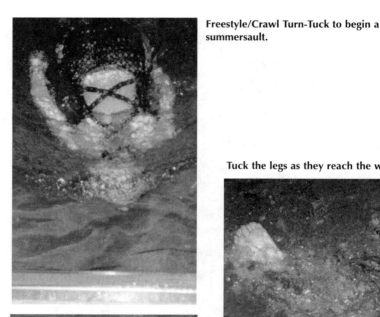

Freestyle/Crawl Turn-Tuck to begin a summersault.

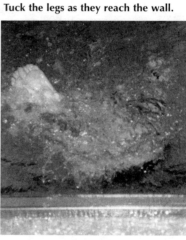

Tuck the legs as they reach the wall.

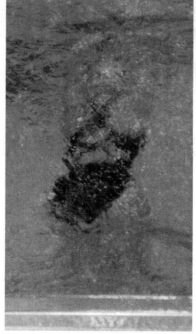

Streamline push off the wall.

COMPETITIVE STARTS

Teach starts in deep water, stressing safety and proper technique.

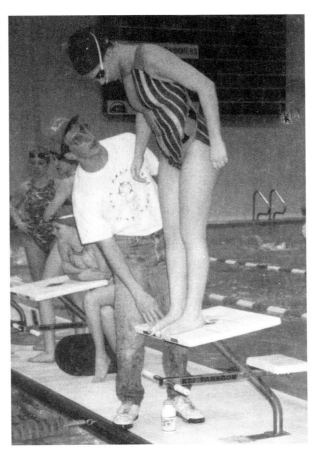

FRONT:
1. Begin start by moving forward, lift head and extend body forward.
2. Streamline body in air.
3. Enter the water and arch your back to reach the surface.

BACKSTROKE STARTS:
1. Begin start by throwing the head back, extending the legs and reach over the head.
2. Arch the back to enter the water, lift the legs during the entry.
3. Dolphin kick to the surface.

Below: Cover starting blocks or limit their access to supervised use only.

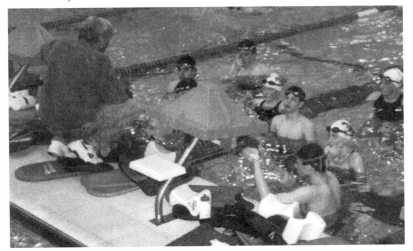

BASIC DIVING

In recent times the incidents of diving accidents has sky rocketed. The importance of learning a dive from the side of a pool can not be over-emphasized.

TEACHING DIVES FROM THE SIDE OF THE POOL SHOULD TAKE PLACE IN WATER AT LEAST 5 FT. DEEP. TALLER, HEAVIER STUDENTS MAY NEED DEEPER WATER.

1. Begin the progression by kneeling on the side of the pool and rolling forward.

2. Next attempt a dive from the side with one leg trailing the other.

Kneeling dive starting position.

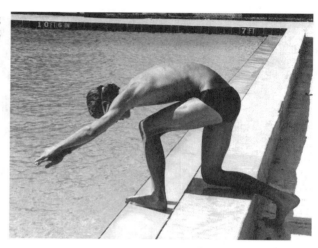

One leg training the other will add a little more momentum when learning a dive.

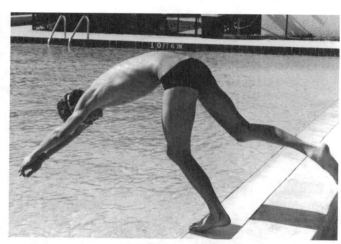

3. Finally, try the standing forward dive.

STUDENTS MAY NEED DEEPER WATER.

Diving should be taught in deep water.

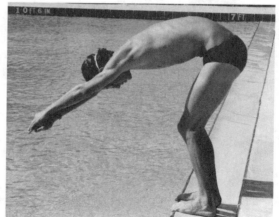

PERSONAL SAFETY

Because swimming takes place in a potentially dangerous medium, water, it is important personal safety dictate the extent to which any activity is pursued in the aquatic environment. The following, are what seem common sense considerations when involved in an activity around the water.

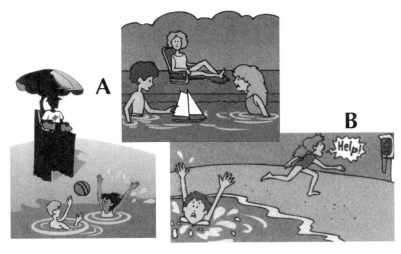

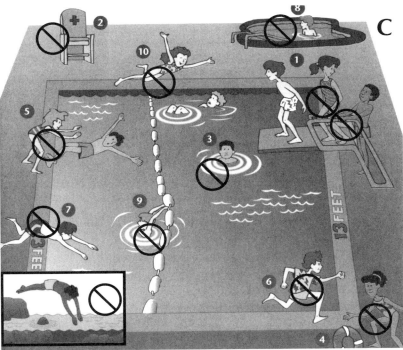

A. Never swim alone, preferably swim in a supervised area.

B. Be aware of your limitations, do not overestimate your ability in water.

C. Be aware of, and follow the rules of a particular aquatic facility. Example rules:
1. Only one diver on the diving board at a time.
2. Make sure there is a lifeguard on duty.
3. Never swim under the diving board.
4. Rescue equipment is for emergencies; leave it in position.
5. Never push someone into the water.
6. Never run on the pool deck.
7. Dive only when you are sure of the depth and condition of the bottom.
8. Even in a pool, never swim alone.
9. Never play on the safety rope.
10. Never jump on or near someone already in the water.

BASIC SAFETY SKILLS

If you plan on spending any time around water, here are some skills that might prove useful in aquatic emergencies. As always, know your limitations and **DO NOT** put yourself at risk.

1. If you see someone in trouble in the water, if possible call for help.

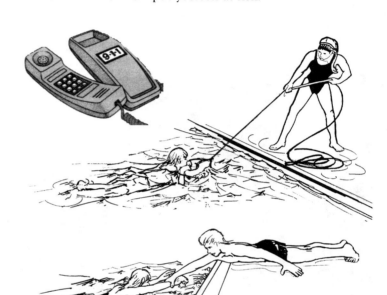

2. The safest way to help a person in trouble is from the side. Reaching, extending or throwing something are the first things you should try.

3. As a last resort enter the water with rescue equipment. Extend the equipment.

   ALWAYS KEEP THE EQUIP-MENT BETWEEN THE VIC-TIM AND YOURSELF.

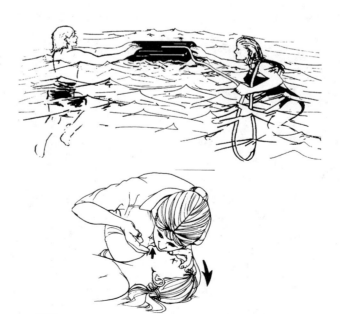

4. Finally, learn CPR and basic First Aid, simply getting the victim out of the water may not be enough.

SAFETY

Aquatic accidents away from man-made aquatic facilities account a large portion of the fatalities associated with water. Here are three areas that must be addressed when looking at total aquatic safety.

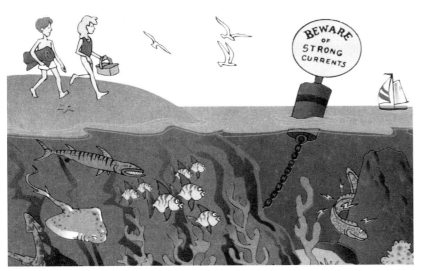

1. Be aware of currents, underwater life, weather conditions and other activities being conducted in the area.

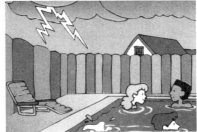

2. Ice, is frozen water. If you find yourself in cold water, remain clothed, try to conserve energy, and slowly attempt to move back to shore. If ice is present, it will be thicker toward the shore line.

3. When boating, make sure P.F.D.'s are present and that they are worn. Additional safety equipment should be on board. If the boat overturns, do not leave it, all approved small craft will float.

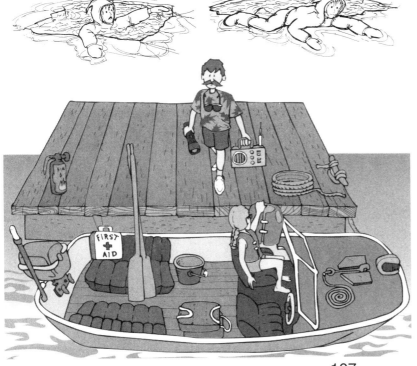

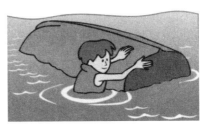

Fitness
WARMING UP

Warming up should be a part of any physical activity. The purpose of the warm-up is to prepare the body for physical activity and prevent possible injury. There are two parts to the warm-up:

1. Slowly elevate the heart rate to about 120 beats per minute.

2. Stretch the muscles to be used in the activity.

1. A simple way to elevate the heart rate is to raise the arms above the head as you inhale and then exhale quickly as the arms are returned to the side.

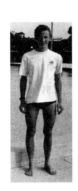 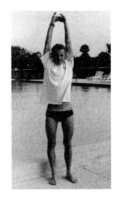 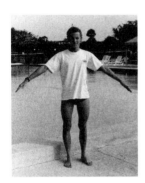 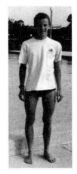

2. Stretching should involve all muscle groups to be used in swimming:

a. Neck circles   **b. Arm stretching**   **c. Arm circles**   **d. Side stretching**   **e. Shoulder circles**

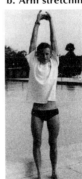 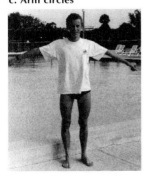 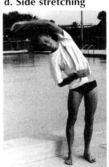 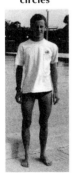

f. Leg stretches   **g. Feet stretching**   **h. Calf stretching**

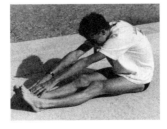 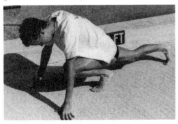 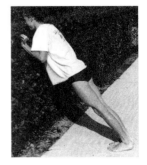

BASIC APPROACH FOR IMPROVEMENT

Improvement in swimming depends on improvement in three areas. They are;
Skill, Endurance, and Speed. Unfortunately, it is next to impossible to maximize training in these three areas at once. Therefore, workouts must target one area without forsaking the other two. In addition, all three areas must be addressed on a regular basis for best results. The following diagrams are suggested as starting points for workouts. Your imagination and work ethic should be your only limiting factor.

MONDAY:

25% Skill	50% Endurance	25% Speed

TUESDAY

33% Skill	33% Endurance	33% Speed

WEDNESDAY

20% Skill	60% Endurance	20% Speed

THURSDAY

33% Skill	33% Endurance	33% Speed

FRIDAY

20% Skill	50% Endurance	30% Speed

Skill training = Drills on specific parts of strokes.
Endurance = Longer distance and moderate speed.
Speed = Shorter distance, more rest

TRAINING DIARY

The following forms are suggestions as to ways to organize your training regiment. Creativity is most important in designing your road to improvement and success.

QUICK DIARY Record total yardage by day and month.

	January	February	March	April	May	June
1						
2						
3						
4						
5						
6						
7						
8						
9						
10						
11						
12						
13						
14						
15						
16						
17						
18						
19						
20						
21						
22						
23						
24						
25						
26						
27						
28						
29						
30						
31						
Total						

	July	August	September	October	November	December
1						
2						
3						
4						
5						
6						
7						
8						
9						
10						
11						
12						
13						
14						
15						
16						
17						
18						
19						
20						
21						
22						
23						
24						
25						
26						
27						
28						
29						
30						
31						
Total						

FULL YEAR TRAINING GRAPH

Record the amount of skill, endurance and speed work completed each week.

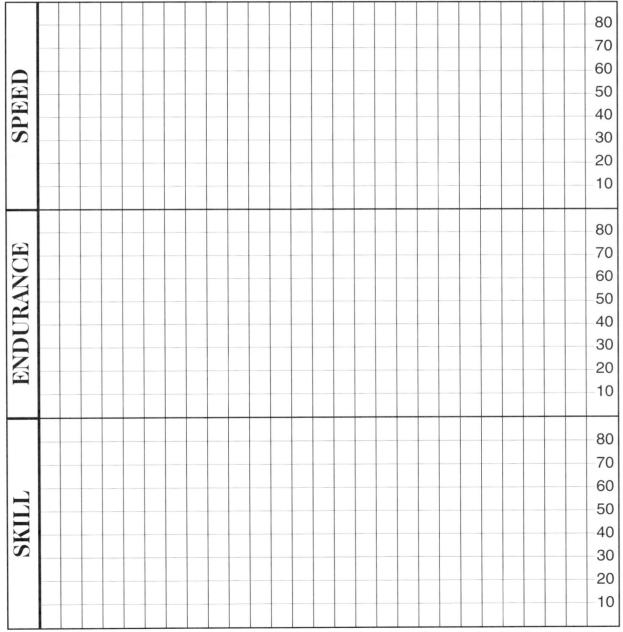

WEEKLY PLAN

MONDAY: Warm-up:

                 Skill set:

                 Endurance set:

                 Speed set:

                 Cool down: Total

TUESDAY: Warm-up:

                 Skill set:

                 Endurance set:

                 Speed set:

                 Cool down: Total

WEDNESDAY: Warm-up:

                 Skill set:

                 Endurance set:

                 Speed set:

                 Cool down: Total

THURSDAY: Warm-up:

                 Skill set:

                 Endurance set:

                 Speed set:

                 Cool down: Total

FRIDAY :   Warm-up:

                 Skill set:

                 Endurance set:

                 Speed set:

                 Cool down:

                                               Total

SAMPLE WORKOUT

Warm-up:	Dry land stretching
	Swim 200 easy any stroke
Skill set:	Drill 12x25's 1-25 kicking
	1-25 arms
	1-25 breathing
	1-25 stroke
Endurance set:	Swim 600 yds (24 lengths) without stopping
	Try to maintain the same pace during the entire swim.
Speed set:	Swim 12x25's fast
	Start every 30 seconds, try to maintain the same pace for each 25.
	*** Note if 30 seconds is too fast, slow it down till you find a
	time you can repeat.
Cool down:	Swim and easy 200 any stroke.
	Total 1600 yds.

SWIMMERS TRAINING FOR THE FIRST TIME MAY WANT TO START OUT WITH MUCH LESS YARDAGE TO BEGIN WITH.

FITNESS CHALLENGE - SWIM THE SEVEN SEAS

Fitness Challenge - Swim the Seven Seas

The Swim The Seven Seas fitness challenge is designed to provide motivation to swimmers who wish to keep track of the yardage swum on a regular basis. The challenge can be tailored to fit three performance levels, for any age:

Novice Seven Seas Challenge- the participant may complete the mileage chart in increments of 100 yard swims.

Advanced Seven Seas Challenge - the participant may complete the mileage chart in increments of 200 yard swims.

Expert Seven Seas Challenge- the participant may complete the mileage chart in increments of 400 yard swims.

Each of the "Seven Seas" is given a mileage requirement, based on it's relative size. Completion awards are given for swimming each `sea' with the final award for completing the 50 miles for all Seven Seas.

Arctic = 10 miles
Antarctic = 20 miles
Indian = 30 miles
N/S Atlantic = 40 miles
N/S Pacific = 50 miles

Swim the Seven Seas personal record cards, wall charts, and award certificates should be used to help swimmers log mileage, provide visibility for the program, and serve as a motivator for both participating and prospective fitness challenge students.

Part 4
Adapted Program

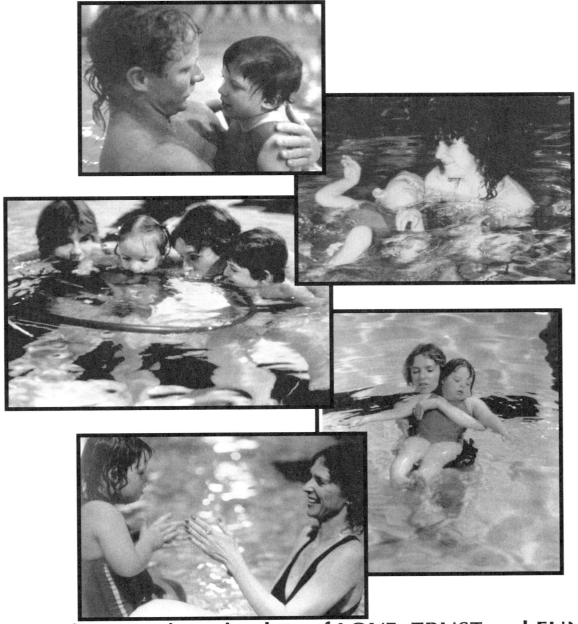

Learning to swim using lots of LOVE, TRUST and FUN!

PROGRAM OVERVIEW

The National Safety Council Adapted Program is administered in conjunction with the Learn to Swim Exploration, Journey, and Challenge components. The licensed Program Coordinator is responsible for quality control, for the safety of participants, and for training instructors. Instructors are trained in how to effectively work with mild to moderately disabled students who may be in any of the Learn to Swim programs.

PROGRAM COORDINATORS
Program coordinators are trained and licensed by Jeff Ellis & Associates, Inc. Coordinators will be held accountable for maintaining the established standard of care and programs will be randomly and independently audited by Jeff Ellis & Associates to ensure compliance. Coordinators conduct instructor training according to their facility needs.

INSTRUCTORS
Instructors may train for, and utilize the Adapted Aquatics course material at the discretion of the Program Coordinator. Time involvement of instructor training can range from 4-8 hours, depending upon experience and needs of the facility. All instructor training must be documented and kept on file.

STUDENTS
Students in the Adapted Aquatics program will have disabilities ranging from mild to moderate, which may effect performance in the water. Students may be enrolled in the Learn to Swim Exploration, Journey, or Challenge programs, or a specialized adapted course may be offered depending upon the programming needs of the facility.

INTRODUCTION

This section is designed to provide additional information regarding teaching swimming to children with mild to moderate disabilities for instructors and program coordinators of the National Safety Council **Learn to Swim Program.** Children who have severe disabilities often require specialized programs, and might not enroll in the **Learn to Swim Program.** However, some may. In fact, this may be the only activity in which they can participate. Many children with disabilities can be included in your classes, and do all the activities described in the Learn to Swim booklets, with little or no adaptation. The child who enrolls in your Learn to Swim Program is, **first and foremost,** a child. Secondly, any child may have some difficulties in performing certain activities. And finally, some children may have specific disabilities which may - **or may not** - affect activity performance. If we focus our attention on the possible cause of performance difficulties - poor balance or coordination, for example - we may be able to help the child do the activities successfully. So, performance factors need to be looked at, rather than types of disability.

Admittedly, there are some factors about disabilities that help one understand performance, so a section about impairments and disabilities has been included. But remember-

For children with mild or moderate disabilities

> First, a child
>
> Second, a child who has varying abilities
>
> Third, a child who has a disability

Most of what you need to know to teach swimming to disabled children you already know— that is, how to teach swimming. Reading this manual will not make you a physical therapist or a recreation therapist. It can, however, help you offer successful and enjoyable learning experiences to children. Swimming is, and always should be, fun— for both the instructor and the student.

Safety must always be your first concern. As in all water-related activities, a lifeguard must be on duty at all times. If the children are very active, inattentive, or not likely to understand or notice safety restrictions, extra lifeguards are needed.

Teaching swimming: fun for the student and fun for the teacher!

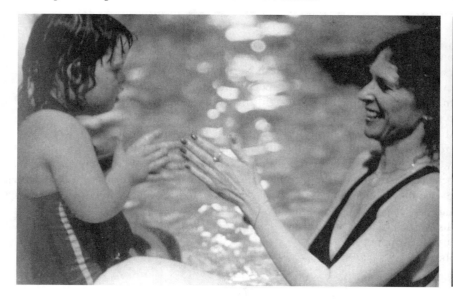

Relating to student

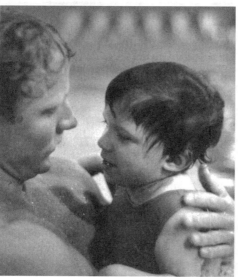

It is great fun to kick and splash!

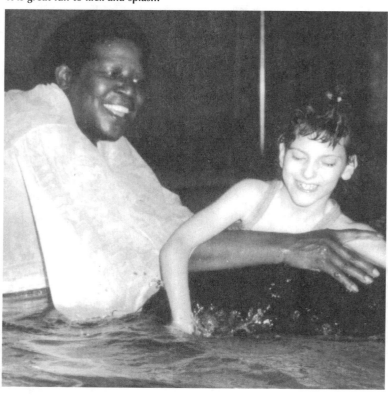

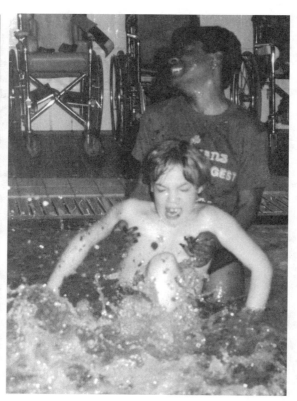

GENERAL PRINCIPLES

Teaching the child with a disability

Teaching children who have disabilities is often no different from teaching those who do not have disabilities. The best teaching is always individualized, as was stated in the Instructor's manual for the National Safety Council Learn to Swim program. The challenge is to adapt teaching methods, and sometimes the skills taught, to each individual participant. For many children with a disability, aquatic activity can be of great benefit in organic development: increasing cardiovascular fitness, muscular strength and endurance, and flexibility. Activities in the water can also be of benefit in perceptual motor development and function, and provide a basis for lifelong participation in a healthful activity. In addition, swimming can provide positive emotional outlets, improved self image, and opportunities for success - all important psychological benefits. There are some social benefits, as well - opportunities for peer interaction, being able to do activities other children do, and learning skills that make the child safer when engaging in recreational activities with family and friends. Most children with disabilities can do the swimming strokes we teach. Instructors should teach correct strokes whenever possible, and modify only if the individual needs to adjust the stroke.

Benefits include: improved fitness, physical strength and endurance.

Other benefits: improved self image, and increased peer interaction.

Your Teaching Approach

Teaching swimming is exciting and fun, and can give lifelong rewards to both swimmers and teachers. Including children with disabilities in your program provides them with experiences and skills they can enjoy, and which can be of great benefit to them; it can also provide you with some wonderful, enriching experiences. Some attributes *that will help you teach children who have disabilities include—*

For the teacher and the student: fun, and lifelong rewards

- **The capacity to care**
  Pablo Casals once said *"The capacity to care is the thing which gives life its greatest significance."* Caring about children is the first ingredient of successful teaching.

- **Knowledge**
  Knowledge of the subject is always important- knowledge of swimming, of child development, and some about disabilities. Do not think, however, that you have to have an advanced degree in rehabilitation to be an effective teacher - you do not. The important thing to remember about knowledge is that sometimes what we know can get in the way of what we could learn. We should always be receptive to new learning.

Don't let what you know interfere with what you can learn.

- **Listening**
  Listening is a skill. Too often, we start thinking about our response - what WE want to say - and forget to listen - to *attend*.

Be open to new knowledge

- **Touch**
  Be understanding about being touched and grabbed - because you probably will be!

- **Your attitudes and prejudices**
  Develop a positive attitude, and throw away your prejudices. Look at the things a child *can* do, not at the things he/she can *not* do. Watch for your own prejudices to surface- you may be surprised at some of the incorrect ideas you retain. (We all do!) Removing prejudice from our own thinking is a lifelong (self-surgery) process.

Learn to LISTEN.

Perhaps the most important thing to remember is that the child with a disability is *first an individual*, then an individual with a disability. Ignore categories and labels— none of us *fits* in a category, or likes to *wear* a label. So, relate to the child as a *child:* one who loves the joy of discovery, a smile of approval, a hug, independence and achievement, just like every child.

If you are uncomfortable, at first, when working with someone who has a disability, don't feel guilty. One new instructor said "I looked at that disabled child, who looked so frail, and I was *sure* that if I picked him up, he'd *break!*" That kind of fear is not unusual. Of course, handling techniques sometimes need to be discussed, and it is appropriate to ask the parent or the child how the child should be picked up, — if *picking up* is necessary. Just remember, this small person is a *person*. Relate to each child as an individual, irrespective of any disability, and establish a relationship of mutual respect and trust. Very soon you will find that uncomfortable feeling going away.

Develop mutual respect and trust

While it is important that you feel comfortable in teaching children who have disabilities, it is also important that a child who has a disability feels comfortable in the learning situation. Many children become more comfortable in the learning environment when expectations are known, the teaching approach is consistent, and communication is effective. This is particularly true of children who have **learning disabilities,** and those who have **behavioral conditions.**

Letting your expectations be known

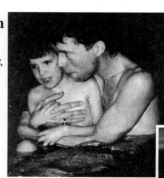

Providing comfort and security

A structured environment, where expectations are known and procedures are the same each day, make it easier for a child to learn and function appropriately. The play environment of the Learn to Swim program may be unstructured, yet there can be aspects of the program which remain the same - taking a shower, sitting in the same place on the deck as the story is read and discussed, entering the pool by the same ladder in the same way, and having the safety rules repeated. The child knows what behaviors are expected, when these things remain predictable.

Active listening.

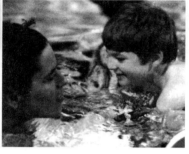

Being consistent in your approach

Give support and comfort. Give a smile.

If you are consistent in your actions and approach, children are more comfortable in the learning environment, and develop trust in you as a teacher. To build that basic trust, you should -

The child has abilities.

- Begin each lesson the same way - use the same procedures each class time.
- Assure the child that you will provide support with your hands and arms when needed
- Always do what you say you will do: if you have promised to support the child while he or she floats, do not take your hands away even if it is apparent that the child is floating independently.
- Set achievable goals, and consult the child for opinion about goals.
- Always remember, the child may have a disability, but also has many abilities. Focus your attention - and the child's - on *abilities and accomplishments.*

Communicating effectively

Listen, attend, pay heed, pay attention, LISTEN.

Effective communication begins with *active listening.* Attending, looking at the speaker, and maintaining eye contact are components of active listening. These actions communicate to the speaker that you are interested and paying attention to what is said. Listening also involves *interpreting* what was said- and responding in a way that helps you know if your interpretation agrees with the speaker's intent.

Developing listening skill is one of the most important aspects of effective communication, and is critical to working with children who may have speech difficulties.

Verbal communication also involves *the words used* - and the *meaning* assigned those words by both the speaker and the listener. Simplifying your vocabulary is often necessary when teaching children, especially those who may have cognitive disabilities. It is still necessary to affirm the child's understanding, by having them tell you what you said, or demonstrate understanding in some way.

Finding help and information

Many knowledgeable people can help you understand performance factors, and aspects of a disability if that is necessary. If you have questions, it is appropriate to ask the child's parents or guardians, teachers, or the child. Several reference books listed in the back of this manual can help expand your knowledge.

If some of the information in this manual is new to you, and you have no experience in working with children who have disabilities, some things you can do to increase your knowledge and your comfort level include—

- Talk to the child. Ask if they have any fears. Ask them what their disability is, and if there are things they shouldn't do.
- Talk to the parents of a child with a disability. They are knowledgeable about their child's disability, and can help you understand. Some may be willing to get in the water and be an aide in the program, and can be most helpful.
- Talk to your Program Coordinator about the possibility of finding a volunteer advisor: someone from a local rehab center or school, who would be willing to observe and advise.
- Observe a classroom or day care program in operation. It is always helpful to observe, before doing something yourself.
- Co-teach with another instructor, especially one who has some experience with children having disabilities.
- Call the office of Ellis & Associates, which keeps a list of people who are willing to answer your questions.
- **Above all,** keep this fact in mind: the best teachers of children with disabilities are those who *care about children,* and are willing to keep learning. You may not know a great deal about various disabilities, but if you....

Those who care about children, and are willing to learn.

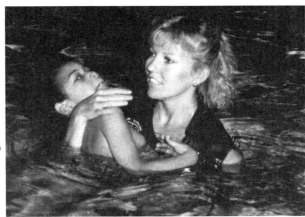

Knowledge and experience will increase your comfort level.

The best teachers care about children, and are willing to keep learning.

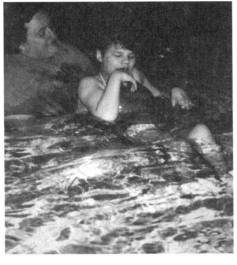

Focus on ABILITY.

..love children,

...are willing to learn from them and from others,

...provide for safety, and

...focus on ability,

you will be a *great success* at teaching swimming to children who have disabilities.

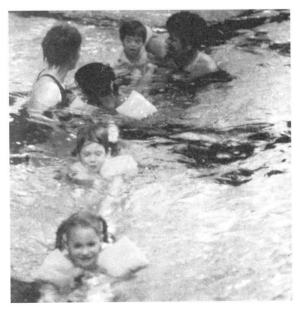

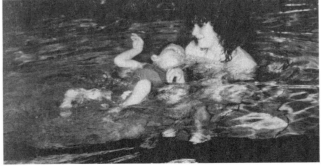

123

FUNCTIONAL FACTORS

Many children who have disabilities can participate in swimming classes, enjoy the **Adventures** with **Swish, Stacey and Jonathan,** and complete the **Journey** with the other children in your class. For some children, teaching may need to be adapted to differences in the way the child is able to move, or the way the child understands. Movement difficulties are often referred to as **motoric** or **motor performance problems,** and are usually due to some impairment in the **perceptual-motor system.** Difficulties in thinking and information processing are usually called **cognitive** problems.

Movement = motoric

Thinking = cognitive

Motor performance

Basically, the perceptual motor system refers to our understanding of sensory input — what the sights and sounds mean to us — and our ability to generate a response. In other words, how we process information and respond to it. We are all perceptual-motor beings, and many children with (and without) disabilities have difficulty with some part of the perceptual-motor process. So, if we look at the different components of perceptual motor performance, we can see things a child might need help with, and figure out how to provide needed help. Components of perceptual motor performance include-

I see or hear-

I understand-

I respond

- balance
- laterality
- visual discrimination
- spatial relationships
- eye-foot coordination

- kinesthetic sense
- directionality
- auditory discrimination
- eye-hand coordination

Observing motor performance

Assessment of perceptual motor performance is not the responsibility of a swimming teacher. However, the following checklist may help in understanding some performance factors which indicate a child may have motoric difficulties. A child *may* have perceptual motor problems if he/she **consistently**

- cannot tell left from right
- cannot move between objects without bumping them
- cannot maintain eye contact with moving objects
- has trouble catching balls or other objects
- cannot hop, or balance on one foot
- cannot identify body parts on command
- seems not to understand directions in space, i.e. up-down; right- left; front- back ; inside-outside.
- seems unable to identify where objects are in relationship to him/ herself in space.

There are other performance factors a classroom teacher or other evaluator might consider, but the preceding list includes those that you might most easily observe when the child is walking on the deck or is in a swimming class. *Occasional poor performance in these areas does not necessarily mean the child has perceptual-motor problems.* The following pages list factors in motor performance, with suggestions for teaching children who may need help in given areas.

Balance — A child who has balance difficulties on land may find balance in the water easier — water is more supportive than air. Thus, you might observe a child coming into your program having difficulty walking on the deck, only to find that the child can walk easily in water! Sometimes, though, various factors can make balance difficult- paralysis, an amputation, or even just a lack of flexibility. Remember, if a child loses balance and cannot regain it without help, that child *must* always have an instructor or aide within arms reach.

Balance: for walking or floating

Counteract imbalance with rotation / counter-balance actions.

In aquatics, balance is needed for walking in water, and for maintaining body position while floating or swimming. The best way to deal with balance problems is to apply principles of *counter-balance*. Counter-balance when walking can be supplied by arm and hand actions, (sculling or finning) : when floating or swimming, counter balance is often supplied by rotation. If the body begins to roll in one direction, rotating the head in the opposite direction often counteracts the roll and provides a return to a balanced position. Raising arms to shoulder level while turning the head increases the counter balance effect.

Buoyancy aids: arm bands, life jackets, buoyancy bars, float mats, bubbles, PFDs and improvised!

If a child is so non-buoyant a stationary float is impossible, momentum often helps that child stay on the surface. So, add a push-off, or a bit of arm or leg action, for momentum. Encourage the child to feel the *sensation* of floating. Sometimes, adding a buoyancy aid at first, (such as air filled arm bands, or foam floats) helps the child understand and **feel** buoyancy. Floatation devices can be gradually removed, or their effect lessened, as the child learns to relax and find the position which keeps him / her afloat.

Most people can easily attain a balanced float, as Gabby Gator explains to Stacey and Jonathan in the *Alligator Alley Adventure* of *Journey 1* ; it is rare, indeed, to find anyone who cannot float in the jellyfish position. Since body configurations differ, assessing buoyancy, balance and other performance factors is very individualized. Do not be hesitant to ask for help, if you have trouble with this. You'll be surprised at how quickly you learn to think of balance, counter-balance, and rotation, and apply principles as necessary.

Kinesthetic Sense — This term means one's ability to sense how the body moves: the direction, extent, and kind of movement of which one is capable. Kinesthetic awareness involves both *body awareness* and *awareness of movement* (locomotor awareness). Locomotor awareness includes awareness of space, of obstacles in space, and how to move around them. Locomotor awareness also involves directionality, discussed later. Many people, - not only some of those who have disabilities - have poor kinesthetic sense.

If a child seems awkward or clumsy, bumping into objects, or cannot follow movement commands with the eyes closed, for example, that child may have a poorly developed kinesthetic sense.

In swimming, kinesthetic sense is important in helping us understand how our arms or legs are moving, as we learn. Most movement activities help develop kinesthetic sense, especially if you and the child both talk about the concept/activity while doing it. The movement chart, Page 11, shows the many ways the body moves.

Laterality — This is the awareness of *sidedness* - left-right; front-back; up-down. If a child does not know left from right, or can't differentiate between left and right, he /she probably has some problems with motor skills involving laterality.

Bilateral action: both sides doing the same thing at the same time.

These laterality skills progress through three levels, each level being more difficult or advanced than the previous level. At the first - bilateral - level, both sides of the body, (both arms, for instance) do the same thing at the same time. This is the easiest type of laterality skill. Examples of this would be-

- holding a kickboard with both hands
- pushing an object with both hands at the same time
- catching a ball with both hands simultaneously
- splashing with both hands simultaneously
- elementary back stroke or breast stroke arm actions

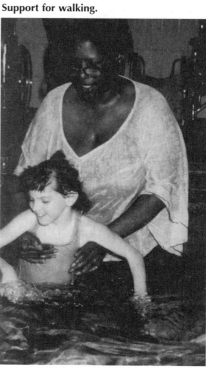
Support for walking.

126

The second level includes activities in which you *alternately* use first one side (arm or leg), and then the other in a cross pattern. These are more difficult than bilateral motions. Examples would be:

Alternating action: first one arm, then the other.

- walking
- climbing
- moving arms in beginner fashion, as Stacey at Seal's Rock
- moving legs alternately, as in the crawl kick

At the highest level, these laterality actions are *integrated* and combine the use of arms and legs and hands in highly organized ways, such as -

1st level: bilateral

2nd level: alternating

3rd level: integrated

- alternating bobbing with throwing or catching activity
- splashing with the hands, while walking
- the crawl stroke. Think about it ! The arms are moving one way, the legs another, the head must turn a specific way, and you also have to remember to breathe correctly! Definitely a skill of high organization.
- other swimming strokes in which arm and leg actions are not in unison: back crawl, butterfly.

Since all of us progress through these levels, it is not unusual to find a child who is developmentally delayed functioning at the first level, and not being able to integrate laterality skills. Children who have mental retardation or developmental delay may need time working on bilateral or alternating skills before integrating skills develop. Activities at the first two levels help the child progress to the third level. Skills in Journey 1 are mostly either bilateral or alternating skills; Journey 2 incorporates more integrated skills.

Directionality

This is laterality in motion — *moving* to the left, or *moving* to the right, moving backwards or forwards, up or down. Many activities and games incorporate directionality skills combined with spatial awareness.

Visual perception

Visual perception is far more than seeing: it involves discriminating between objects, and correctly interpreting and responding to that which is seen. (Examples of discrimination tasks would be choosing correctly between a round object and a square object, correctly perceiving the depth of the pool, or differentiating between something floating and something on the bottom of the pool.)

Seeing
- discriminating
- interpreting
- responding.

Poor visual perception is not the result of poor visual acuity, but rather a function of processing in the brain. It is an inability to interpret accurately what the eyes see, or inability to respond.

In addition to discrimination tasks, visual perception includes responses involved in eye-hand coordination, and eye-foot coordination. Thus, a child who cannot catch a ball, or find and retrieve an object, or step over an obstacle, may have a visual perception problem.

Many children who have a developmental delay, or who have mental retardation, have eye-hand or eye-foot coordination difficulties.

Auditory Perception

Auditory perception involves ability to interpret sounds, translate them into information, and respond. This involves listening skills, language reception, following directions, and rhythmic movement. Clapping to music, and responding in games like musical hula hoops and whistle tag are auditory discrimination activities.

Hearing
- discriminating
- interpreting
- responding.

Children who have hearing impairments may have trouble in this area because of limited input, but poor auditory response is not due to poor auditory acuity, but rather is a function of processing in the brain.

Spatial Awareness

Spatial awareness is understanding of *self space* (space the body occupies), and location of one's body in *general* space. Visual and kinesthetic feedback during movement greatly affect one's spatial awareness.

Sometimes, children with poor spatial awareness have trouble perceiving where the bottom of the pool is, and may be hesitant to jump into the pool. They may also be unsure of the location of other swimmers in the pool, or of objects floating or on the bottom of the pool. Activities involving spatial awareness can include games like musical hula hoops, a water obstacle course, exchange tag, and jumping off of Seals Rock in Adventure 1.

Eye-hand Coordination

Eye-hand coordination is control of hand movements by visual guidance. All catching, throwing and retrieval activities require eye-hand coordination. Ball games, tag games, and retrieval relays are examples.

Visual discrimination, kinesthetic awareness and space perception also play a part in eye-hand coordination.

Eye-foot coordination

Eye-foot coordination is control of foot movement by visual guidance. Activities involving eye-foot coordination are things like walking on a line, walking in a prescribed space or pattern, kicking a ball, or stepping over obstacles.

Activities and games involving these factors of perceptual-motor development can increase abilities of children who exhibit functional deficits in these areas. Self confidence and independence in movement can be ultimate results. Since the activities are developmental in nature, and thus applicable to all children, they are especially useful in mainstream or inclusive programs.

The following three pages contain a summary of the preceding information on perceptual motor function, and some suggested activities designed to help you apply these principles to your teaching in aquatics.

MOVEMENT CHART

SPACE AWARENESS

WAYS THE BODY USES SPACE

Directions	Levels	Pathways	Ranges
Forward	High	Straight	Large
Backward	Medium	Curved	
Medium			
Sideways	Low	Zigzag	Small
Left			
Right			
Up			
Down			

BODY AWARENESS

WHAT THE BODY IS	WHAT THE BODY DOES
Body Parts	**What the body parts can do**
Head,neck	Support
Arms,legs	Lead
Trunk,hands,feet	Transfer weight
Body Surfaces	**Shapes the Body can Make**
Front	Round, Curled
Back	Straight, Long
Sides	Narrow, Stretched
	Symmetrical, Asymmetrical

RELATIONSHIPS

RELATIONSHIP OF THE BODY TO OBJECTS, INDIVIDUALS, GROUPS

	Near
	Far
	Meeting
	Parting
	Surrounding
	Above
Body parts to body parts	Beneath
Individuals to groups	Alongside
Body parts to objects	In front of
Groups to objects	Behind
	Across
	Leading
	Following
	Mirroring
	Shadowing
	Unison
	Contrast

BASIC MOVEMENTS THE BODY CAN MAKE

Locomotor	Manipulative	Nonlocomotor	Maneuver Weight
Walk, run	Kick	Bend, stretch	Push, pull
Jump, hop	Strike	Curl, twist	Lift, carry
Leap, gallop	Throw	Turn, swing	Resist, receive
Skip, slide	Catch	Sway	Support, initiate
			Transfer

QUALITY OF BODY MOVEMENT

HOW THE BODY MOVES

In Time	With Force	In Space	With Flow
Fast	Strong-weak	Direct	Bound
Slow	Heavy-light	Flexible	Free
Accelerating	Relaxed		Sequential
Decelerating	Created-absorbed		Continuous
			Broken

Every Child a Winner Lesson Plans, 1987
Reproduced by permission of the authors,
Martha Owens and Susan Rockett.

TEACHING FOR PERCEPTUAL MOTOR PERFORMANCE

Children with perceptual-motor deficits can have many difficulties in the aquatic environment. A child with poor spatial orientation may have difficulty in perceiving the location of people and things in relation to him/herself, and may be unable to perceive the depth of the water or distance to the wall accurately. Each of the components of perceptual-motor performance can affect a child in the water in many ways.

Components of perceptual motor learning:

- Balance
- Visual discrimination
- Auditory discrimination
- Eye-hand coordination
- Eye-foot coordination

- Kinesthetic sense
- Laterality
- Directionality
- Spatial relationships

Studies have shown that a well planned physical activity program can contribute to motor development. Teaching for perceptual motor performance can be effective in aquatic programs which include children with and without disability. The activities become therapeutic for the child with a disability, and are developmental for the child who has no disability. One possible plan, or model, is below.

P/M factor	Skill/activity	Swim level	Pool area	Equip.	Fun

Choosing the component of perceptual motor function that needs development/remediation, the teacher (1) decides upon skills, games, or activities which utilize that function, (2) considers the aquatic level of the students, (3) decides on appropriate pool area to use or modify, (4) selects appropriate equipment, and (5) figures out ways to make it all enjoyable.

Plan a class activity for each factor of perceptual-motor performance.

Perceptual-motor Performance

Operational definition: Perceptual motor performance is a chain of events which begins with a sensory stimulus, goes through a cognitive process, and elicits a motoric response.

Input	Process	Output
Sensory Stimulus	Cognitive process	Motor response
See	Know	Do

In almost all disabilities, there is *some* deficit in *some* part of that process.

Disabilities and the location of impairment in the information processing system

Perceptual motor Process

Disability	Input	Process	Output
Visual	-	+	+
Hearing	-	+	+
Learning	+	-	+ /-
M R	+	-	+ /-
C P	+	+ (-)	-
Orthop.	+	+	-

- A minus sign designates a disablement
+ A plus sign designates lack of disablement

The above is not a model of perceptual motor learning, since it leaves out some critical aspects such as feedback, practice and motor planning. It does illustrate that many disabled children have perceptual motor problems.

Worksheet

Performance component	Description	Activity
Balance	Ability to maintain equilibrium	Counter-balance, rotation
Laterality	Awareness of right and left	Bilateral & alternating activity
Visual discrimination	Seeing, interpreting, responding	Identify objects, shapes
Spatial relationships	Location of self/ things in space	Water obstacle course
Kinesthetic sense	Awareness of type of movement	Arm & leg movements
Directionality	Specific movement	Move right/left, up/down
Auditory discrimination	Interpreting/responding to sound	Musical hula hoops
Eye-hand coordination	Visual control of hand movement	Tag, pick-up games
Eye-foot coordination	Visual control of foot movement	Walking a line, around objects

Components of perceptual motor performance are listed in the first column. They are described in the second column. The third column lists an activity which utilizes the component. In the activity (third) column, **list at least two more activities** for each component.

FUNCTIONAL FACTORS - COGNITIVE

Cognitive Function

Cognitive function refers to the way we *process information* — our understanding of information received, and our ability to plan and execute a response. There is great variation in this process: some people process information very rapidly, some much less rapidly.

Some things affecting our cognitive functioning include —
- basic intelligence
- previous learning / experience
- meaningfulness of the material or action

Understanding - planning - responding.

If a child in your Learn to Swim program seems to have trouble understanding, or is very slow to respond, the child **may** have a cognitive function impairment. There are various things you as a teacher can do, to help a child understand.

Simplifying your vocabulary — Use words you believe the child understands, and try expressing the same information in several ways. Learn to be verbally simple but not talk down to a student.

Keep the words simple.

Simplifying the actions requested — It is not unusual for individuals who have cognitive impairments to have difficulty with *sequencing*, or following directives with several components. Using single concept or action commands makes it easier for a child to understand.

For instance, telling a child to "swim through the hula hoop" involves only one movement concept, the concept of *through*. However, telling the child to "swim over, under, around and through the hoop" requires that the child not only understand all of those concepts, but be able to do them in the sequence asked.

One step at a time.

Using repetition — Repeating activities helps with memory: it reinforces the concept or information learned. Repeating activities during a lesson, and reviewing past activities helps the child remember. Repetition need not be boring — it might include doing the same skill in a different way, or doing the same skill but describing it differently.

Repeat and review.

Providing specific feedback — Praise for a job well done is important to all of us, but in motor learning, the praise must be *immediate* and very *specific*. If a skill has several components, it must often be taught one component at a time, especially if the child has a cognitive function deficit. Specific praise provides the child with knowledge that the skill (or the component) has been done correctly.

Quick praise for specific actions.

Verifying the child's understanding — We should do this in all teaching, but it is of particular importance when teaching children who may have cognitive function deficits. It is not enough to accept the child's nod of assent when you have asked if he or she understands. You should have the child show by some action that he or she does indeed understand the directive.

Understanding components of motor performance and cognitive functioning can help you adapt teaching methods, and give help in specific areas when needed.

There are several reasons for the emphasis on function, in the preceding pages. Increased function can provide bridges to independence, to health, to family activities and shared experiences, and to healthful, lifelong recreation. A child who can swim is much safer in a family boating activity, or a camping outing. A child who has an increased range of motion and ability to move can function independently in many ways, improving the self concept and changing family interactions in positive ways. Just placing the emphasis upon function removes the emphasis on disability — helps remove the label which can be a stigma.

Have fun and be safe.

Even as we look at function, we need to do so positively, looking at what the child can do, not what he or she cannot do. Labeling creates walls, focusing on abilities creates bridges. Looking at perceptual motor function helps us focus our attention on similarities rather than differences. Increasing perceptual motor function helps the child be like, and perform like, peers who do not have a disability. As a teacher of swimming, you are trained to look at function, and looking at function shows you the things upon which you can have impact; ways you can help children.

Lastly, increased function in these areas help children learn to swim and have greater enjoyment in the water. People swim to have fun; providing children with swimming skill opens the door to experiences and fun not previously available to them. As a swimming teacher, you are opening the door to the possibility of lifelong fun and enjoyment in the water. Aquatic activity is a path to function and fun.

Getting accustomed to water

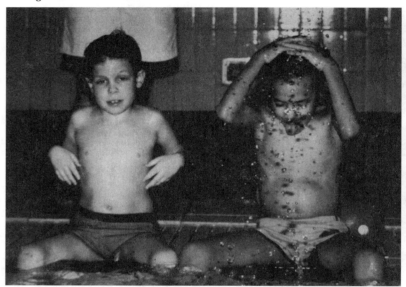
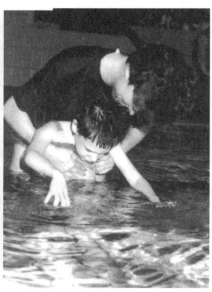
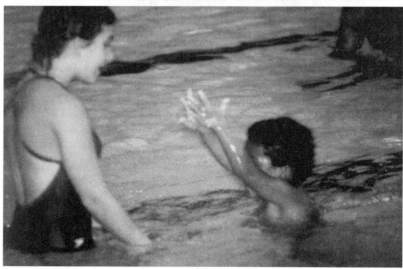

DISABILITIES

This section deals with some disabilities, and ways they might affect a child's performance in the water. Obviously, all disabilities cannot be covered, nor is it necessary - we deal with disabilities which are most common, and which children who come to your program might have. In many instances, you may not even know a child has a disability, but may observe performance factors, and be able to use information in Section I of this manual, to adapt teaching methods.

Additional information sources are listed in the reference section in the back of this manual. Remember, children and their parents may be your best information sources.

Cerebral Palsy

Cerebral palsy is a congenital impairment of the central nervous system causing loss of voluntary muscle control. Cerebral palsy is greatly variable — effect on function may range from very mild to very severe. If involvement is minimal, the child may have only mild problems with motor control, or may have only slight impairment of function on one side of the body. A child with more severe cerebral palsy may have jerky or uncertain, purposeless movements, contracted muscles, speech and breathing difficulties, and may lack ability to control head position.

CEREBRAL PALSY - contracted muscles, speech and balance difficulty, breath control problems, minimal head control and flexibility

Children who are severely involved may have almost a tuck body position, caused by extreme hip flexion. They may also have a tonic neck thrust caused by tension (extra tone) of the neck muscles. This added tonicity may cause lifting of the chin and a semifixed head position. In the prone position, the head and neck may thrust upward. In the supine position, the child may hyperextend the head backwards into the water, and may need constant support when in this position. Some individuals have a "startle reflex", a spastic muscle response to sudden, loud noises.

Warm water (84-94 degrees F.) facilitates relaxation, and is generally preferred for beginners who have cerebral palsy. Individuals who have severe cerebral palsy often cannot walk, and use wheelchairs for mobility on land. Often, even non-buoyant children who have learned to be comfortable in water can achieve independent mobility in aquatic activities.

Aquatic activities build strength and endurance.

If a child's general physical fitness level is low, the gradual increase of activity may help build greater strength and endurance, both of which are vitally important to health and independent functioning.

Most individuals with cerebral palsy are not mentally retarded, but, unfortunately, people often make that assumption based upon the individual's difficulties in speech or lack of speech, and other physical characteristics. Remember, your best information source about the child may be the child, or perhaps his/her parent, guardian or care-taker. It is appropriate to ask about function, for safety's sake. It is also appropriate to ask for a word or sentence to be repeated, if the child's speech is difficult to understand. *Never* pretend to understand - always ask that the words be repeated, or the sentence said a different way.

It's okay to ask.

Many children and adults who have cerebral palsy become very good swimmers, and enjoy aquatic competition at national and international levels.

Effect on Aquatic Participation

Because of involvement of face and neck muscles, a child with cerebral palsy may have difficulty controlling breathing, and, in fact, may not be able to close the air passage and submerge the face. So one of the first tasks of an instructor, after getting the child into the pool, should be to determine the child's ability to control breathing and head position. The upright position is usually more restful, for a child with severe cerebral palsy, than is either the prone or supine position. Independent walking in water is excellent activity, and can

Independent walking - an exciting achievement

be an exciting achievement for individuals who have limited mobility on land. Most individuals who have cerebral palsy are non-buoyant, and may need buoyancy aids to achieve floating and mobility skills. When teaching children who have cerebral palsy, there are two primary areas of concern - amount of movement capability, and ability of the child to hold his/her breath.

Teaching Suggestions

- Help children understand the supportive nature of water. When standing or walking, they should be in chest deep water, and learn to use the hands for balance by moving them back and forth in the water (sculling or finning).

- For a severely involved child, the vertical position can usually be considered a resting position. A child with severe cerebral palsy should be supported in this upright position, (by holding the waist or under the arms) while you determine amount of head control.

Support and watch the child's head

- Be especially careful at first, to avoid any incidents that might cause fear. Remain at the child's head, where he/she can see you. Support the child's head, and watch for sudden reflexive movements that might cause the head to submerge.

- A back float (supine) position allows for ease of breathing, and should usually follow water orientation in the upright position.

- Children who have flexed arms attain mobility more easily in the prone position, but this position cannot safely be used until you are sure of a child's ability to control both breathing and head position.

Use your shoulder as a pillow

- When first helping a child to a supine position, the best method is to have the student's head resting on your shoulder, with your hands supporting the student's lower back. (Adjust your body position - bend your knees - so that your shoulder is at water level.) Later you may be able to move to an alternative position, in which you hold under the child's arms, and let your forearms support the child's head.

- Extreme tension (hypertonicity) of arm muscles may cause a child's arms to stay bent (flexed) at all times. Never apply pressure to try to straighten (extend) the arm. However, warm water and gentle activity may help a child extend his/her reach. As children learn swimming skills, they should be encouraged to extend and use as much range of motion as possible.

Develop a signal for emergencies

- If a child's speech is difficult to understand, ask that the statement be repeated, or said in a different way. Each child has a slightly different speech pattern, and if you listen carefully, you will soon learn to understand much of what the child is saying. **You should use or develop an emergency signal a student in trouble can quickly convey.**

- If a child is non buoyant, flotation devices may be used on both the upper body and legs. (They should never be used on the legs unless the upper body is also supported with flotation.) Remember, a child using flotation devices should never be left alone in the water.

- Any adaptation which helps a child achieve independent mobility should be used; in fact, independent mobility may be a primary goal.

- If you carefully observe a child's range of motion, you may easily find alternative ways for him/her to participate in an Adventure with Swish. Many children with cerebral palsy can participate in all aspects of the Adventures, and will not require extra help.

Modeling: moving the child's legs in the desired pattern of motion.

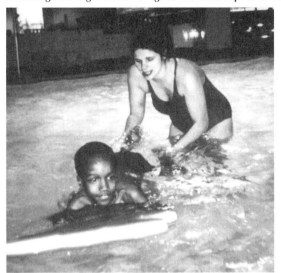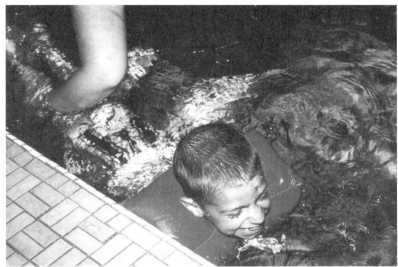

Flotation devices help with water adjustment.

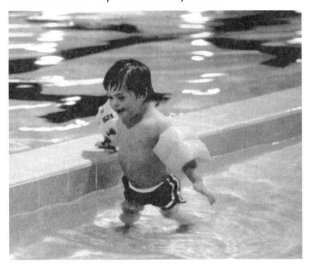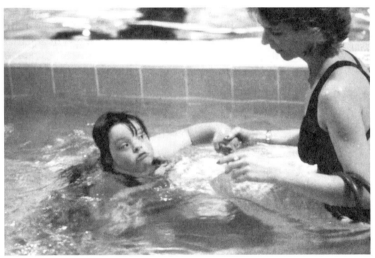

Toys and equipment help make it fun.

EMOTIONAL/BEHAVIORAL DISORDERS

Behavioral Disabilities

Child may dislike change.

Behavioral disabilities - sometimes referred to as emotional disturbance - are disturbances in behavior and emotional reactions, of marked degree and over a considerable period of time. Children who have mild to moderate behavior disabilities are usually mainstreamed in our society. A child who has a behavioral disability may be verbally and physically aggressive and disruptive, or may appear withdrawn, excessively shy, and extremely anxious. Barriers to achievement may cause the child to blame others, withdraw, or become aggressive.

Let the child know what you expect.

The child's responses may be unpredictable and variable, and he/she may strongly object to *any change* in routine or in the environment. Situations which cause stress and fear should be avoided. Safety rules may need to be repeated often. It is best to have the same teacher work with the group each lesson. Children who have behavioral disabilities function best when expectations are known, the teaching approach is consistent, and communication is effective.

Effect on Aquatic Participation

Give specific feedback: tell the child what was done well

Behavioral conditions affect children's participation in social interactions and group situations, and the teacher's class control and teaching methods in aquatics. Special attention must be given to providing positive reinforcement, a structured environment and extra time for adjustment to the water and new situations. The simple activities in the Learn to Swim Program, and the play approach, may be easier for children who have behavioral conditions than complex games or even games of low organization.

A child who has a behavioral condition may ignore safety rules — extra lifeguards and regular reminders may be needed.

Teaching Suggestions

- Teach skills in increments if necessary, and provide feedback immediately.
- Lessons should provide opportunities for success — and successful completion of tasks should be rewarded with immediate positive feed-back.

Build a relationship with the child.

Let the child know you care.

- Establish a personal relationship with children who have behavioral disabilities - having the same instructor for each class facilitates establishing a relationship, and also accommodates the child's dislike of change.
- An atmosphere of caring is essential. Show the child you care about him/her by learning the child's name immediately, by eye contact and smiling, and by enthusiastic responses to successful achievement.
- Children with behavior disabilities may respond well to use of toys and equipment, and may relate to the toy rather than to the teacher or other children. Use toys - and share toy use with a child - to facilitate personal interactions.
- Aggressive behavior may need to be controlled - however, varying the activities will often stop aggressive behavior.

Hearing Impairments

Hearing impairments have great variation - a mild hearing loss might make little difference in a child's functional ability. If the child has a moderate loss, normal conversation might be perceived as a whisper.

Face the child - speak normally.

Individuals with profound hearing losses perceive only very loud sounds, probably wear hearing aids, and use manual communication along with speech reading. Most hearing impairments are congenital - the child is born with that condition.

Generally speaking, a hearing impairment does not affect the child adversely in learning to swim — it is your ability to communicate with the child that may be challenging. If the child speech-reads (lip-reads), it is important to face the child when speaking, and not over-exaggerate lip movements. In other words, speak normally.

However, since less than one third of speech sounds in the English language can be visually discerned, you cannot rely on speech reading to provide a child with all needed information. Therefore, demonstrations are important. Deaf children are usually very visual - they are used to relying on visual input, so they watch carefully.

If a child uses manual communication (sign language), you should make the effort to learn several basic signs: Watch me. Good. Jump. Stop. Toilet. The child will probably love to teach you a few signs.

Effect on Aquatic Participation

A hearing impairment may have almost no effect on a child's participation in a swimming class. Watching other children, a deaf child may simply imitate what they are doing. You may need to call attention to specific pictures in the Learn to Swim book, and explain what Stacey and Jonathan are doing. Enlist the help of the child's parent - reading about the activities when they are at home increases a child's understanding.

Generally speaking, careful and thoughtful orientation to the pool and the first experiences in the water provide a base for the child's full participation in the swimming program.

Some children wear ear molds while swimming. These are individually designed, and the child (or parent) knows if they are to be worn. Children who wear ear molds or ear plugs should not jump into or dive into the water. If the child usually wears a hearing aid, taking it off, to swim, greatly changes sensory input. Many children do not wish to give up hearing aids to enter the water. Be especially reassuring at first; a smile, and saying (and signing) "It's ok," and "Watch me" will probably help.

Teaching Suggestions

- Make sure the student watches you when you speak or demonstrate a skill. It is often more effective to have another student demonstrate, so you may sign "Watch," point to the other student, and have them demonstrate. Even better - if the child with a disability learns a skill before a non-disabled child, let the child with a disability demonstrate.
- Moving a child's arms or legs in a desired pattern of movement helps the child understand, and enhances kinesthetic awareness.
- Use pictures in the Learn to Swim books to help explain what it is you want the child to do.
- Teach the child to keep the eyes open, both above and under water. Visual input is extremely important to a child with a hearing impairment.
- If a child seems not to have a complete understanding of space and depth, use many ways of explaining and showing distance and depth. Practice concepts of far, near, up and down, and have the child demonstrate his/her understanding.
- If the child's speech is difficult to understand, practice your own listening skills, and learn the meaning of the verbalized sounds.
- It is sometimes advisable to have extra safety spotters on deck in addition to the regular lifeguard, especially if there are problems with communication.
- Devise a signal system which you can use in emergencies, to replace whistles and other auditory signals.

Learning Disabilities

A learning disability is a permanent condition which affects ways a person of average or above average intelligence takes in and processes information. Learning disabilities are often specific, in that they affect only one part of learning or functioning - the ability to read, for example. Some children who have a learning disability have perceptual motor difficulties (see pgs. 125-132) and benefit from activities enhancing balance, space perception, coordination, etc. Some are hyperactive and seem to have a short attention span; some

Learn some signs

Look / watch

Shower

Careful

Thank you

Good

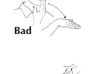
Bad

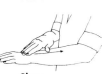
Walk

Slow

Practice active listening

Child may be hyperactive, and may have a short attention span.

may appear to be highly emotional. Sometimes, children who are learning disabled continue a behavior or an activity, and seem to be unable to stop. (This is called perseverating.) If a child perseverates, it may be necessary to stop the behavior physically, give the instruction again, and physically stop the behavior at the appropriate place or time.

Children who have learning disabilities function best in a structured environment, where expectations are known and events predictable. Reading the Learn to Swim Journey books helps make events predictable. Retaining the attention of a distractible child can be a challenge - varying activities and using activities which the child enjoys (and at which the child is successful) can help you do this.

Most children who have a learning disability are able to function with non-disabled children in the Journeys, and enjoy the Adventures with Swish, Stacey and Jonathan, with only a small amount of additional help from you.

Effect on Aquatic Participation

Initial sessions, and adjustment to the water, are of special importance. Generally speaking, a child who has difficulty with space perception may have no concept of depth of the water, and may have difficulty judging distance from the wall or from other swimmers. The child may have difficulty adjusting to new visual cues when changing positions in the water - from upright to back position, for instance. The child may also understand a demonstration or explanation, and still be unable to act upon that understanding, due to a perceptual motor problem. Actually moving the child's arms, legs, or total body through an activity can help the child understand the activity. It is also useful to have a child feel your arm as it moves in a desired pattern. (This is called co-action, or coactive modeling.)

Extra security may be necessary to the child at first - you may need to hold the child, or hold his /her hand at first, as you go through Adventures.

Teaching Suggestions

- Provide security if the child is afraid or extremely insecure in the environment.
- Some children need multisensory cues and instructions — say what you want the child to see, point to it, and place the child's hand on the object discussed. A multisensory cue about Under the Sea in Adventure 1, for instance, might involve you talking about Jonathan's humming, pointing to the picture in the child's book, humming yourself, having the child point to Jonathan, and asking the child to hum.
- Multisensory cues help most children learn, so are good teaching techniques for your classes.
- If a child has obvious space perception problems, it is best to provide good visual references in initial pool experiences. Usually, that means your face should be in front of the child, until he/she is comfortable with the wider vista of the pool. Your smiling face, of course!
- Reducing perceived space seems to help some children deal with new and large environments, like a swimming pool. Several things can do this — your outstretched arms, buoy lines, strategically placed equipment.
- Consistency is important; use the same words each time you want a specific response.
- Seeing someone float in a demonstration, or reading about Stacey and Jonathan in Alligator Alley, may not prepare a child for the feeling of buoyancy. Be ready to provide secure support as the child floats and/or attempts to stand up (do a recovery) after floating.
- A child who has poor spatial perception may have difficulty understanding the concept of *space behind*, and thus be reluctant to assume a back float position. Give extra support (holding), and talk about the differences in the visual field (different things the child sees).
- If a child is hyperactive and distractible, minimizing noise and outside distractions is advisable. A calm voice and firm (but smiling) approach from the teacher are helpful.
- New environments can be frightening. Be extra reassuring and supportive during initial lessons. Although security and support are stressed here, and often needed, the goal for the child is independent functioning. Gradually move the child to independence, and reinforce independent activity with a smile and a "Well done!".

We can have the fun of swimming in the water

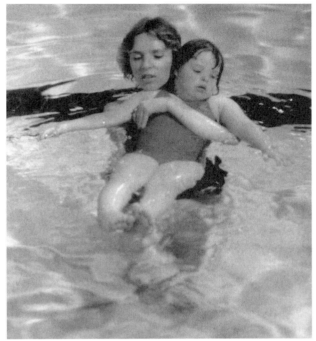

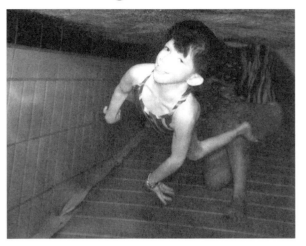

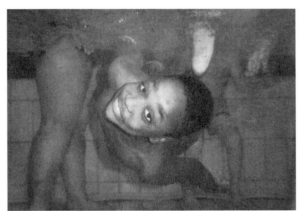

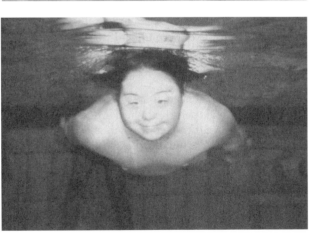

Mental Retardation

Mental retardation is a condition existing at birth, often from unknown causes. There are other terms used, such as cognitive disability and developmental delay. Sometimes there are associated physical characteristics, as in Down syndrome. There are levels of retardation - mild, moderate, severe/profound. Most people with mental retardation are more like than unlike their peers who are not retarded . In other words, there are more similarities than there are differences.

The most common characteristic of children who have mental retardation is slowness in learning. Often, teachers must segment skills - teach only one part at a time - and use more than the usual repetition and review. Some children (and adults) do have poor motor coordination, and some may be in poor physical condition from lack of exercise; water play can provide much-needed activity.

Some children may have short attention spans. Short, simple explanations help retain the child's attention, and aid in understanding. Many children can function very well with no special help in a regular swimming class.

Effect on Aquatic Participation

Fear of new situations may sometimes cause a child to appear stubborn or aggressive. It may be necessary to spend extra time on water adjustment, although the play and adventure approach of the Learn to Swim Program may make water adjustment easy. Some children show no fear, and may lack judgement regarding water depth. Providing security and adequate support in initial experiences reduces anxieties. If the children are also hyperactive, extra lifeguards are needed. If a child has poor coordination and motor ability, activities may need to be repeated and reviewed.

Teaching Suggestions

- Keep explanations simple and concise — use the KISS - MIF approach. (Keep It Super Simple - Make It Fun)
- If a child does not seem to understand an explanation, try moving the child's arms or legs in the desired pattern of movement. Manually guiding the child's arms or legs is often more effective than verbal explanations.
- Praise should be specific - not just "Good!" but "Good, you moved your arm down!"
- Sequencing may be difficult for some children; they may not be able to follow instructions which give them two or three things to do in sequence. Teach skills and activities as simple components, not complex combinations.
- If a child is self-abusive — bites himself/herself, or hits his/her head against a wall — ask for guidance from the parent or other care-taker about appropriate ways to deal with the behavior. (You should use the techniques they use.) Varying activities and offering reassurance often reduces self abusive behavior.
- It is important to not talk down to students - do not talk to a 12 year old as if he/she were only 3 years old. Use age-appropriate vocabulary.
- Encourage the child to talk about what he/she is doing in water; verbalization helps learning. If the child is not very verbal, then talk about activities while they are being done. This parallel talk also aids understanding and promotes speech.
- Breath control and bubble blowing help the child with both water adjustment and speech development.
- Some children have no fear of the water, and may behave in dangerous ways. Be especially aware of safety needs, and observe the child at all times. Never turn your back on children in your class.
- Many children who are mentally retarded have a lag in motor development, and may not be in good physical condition. Their rates of progress in motor development skills may be slower than some other students.

Keep explanations short and simple.

The three R's:

Reassurance, Repetition, Review

One step at a time

Parallel talk: talk about the activity while doing it.

Safety ALWAYS

Muscular Dystrophy

Muscular dystrophy is a progressive disease of the muscles, more often affecting boys than girls. It first affects the hip girdle muscles, causing difficulty in walking and climbing steps, and may have associated general weakness. Balance and muscular strength and endurance are usually reduced.

Difficulties in walking and climbing.

Although physical activity will not restore deteriorated muscles, such activity can enhance adjacent muscles, help to retain function, and slow the progressive nature of the condition. Warm water is desirable; cold water may increase muscle cramping and inhibit relaxation.

Effect on Aquatic Participation

General weakness and progressive nature of muscular dystrophy affect both rate of skill acquisition and retention of acquired skills. Muscles of the chest are involved at some point in the disease's progression, so respiration may be difficult or impaired. However, aquatic activities can help retain strength and function, and are usually considered very beneficial.

Encourage independent action.

Ongoing assessment of functional abilities and revision of goals are essential in a progressive condition such as muscular dystrophy.

Teaching Suggestions

- Maintaining independent action is important; do not help with an action a child can do alone
- Do not allow the student to overexert and become fatigued. Keep activities enjoyable, lessons short, and watch the child for signs of fatigue.
- Floating, turning over to a back float, and finning with the hands are important skills to teach.
- Use your hands to support the child in first attempts at floating; maintain that support as the child learns to recover (stand) from the float — recovery may be more difficult than the float.
- Explain mechanics of the recovery to the child, so the importance of the sequence is understood —

Recovery from the back float

1. Drop the hips to a sit position
2. Scull with the hands
3. Put the feet down on the floor of the pool
4. Lift the head
5. Come to an upright stance

Independent mobility. Exercise and fun.

Recovery from the front float

1. Tuck
2. Push down with hands
3. Put the feet down on the floor of the pool
4. Lift the head
5. Come to an upright stance

- Modify strokes as necessary — stylized swimming is not nearly so important as independent mobility, exercise, and fun.
- Shoulder girdle weakness may allow the child to slip through or off a flotation device that is not well secured. Carefully observe and monitor children when using flotation aids.
- Encourage the child in independent action as long as it is possible. Activity helps retain function as the disease progresses.
- Usually, function of arm muscles is retained much longer than that of leg muscles, so it is important to teach activities which can be done with mostly arm muscles - back float with arm action close to the sides, for instance. (Stacey and Jonathan do this in Journey 1.)
- As the disease progresses, walking balance and safe methods of pool entry also change. Lack of muscle strength may make it impossible for the child to help himself/herself if starting to fall. Stay close to

Teach back float with arm or hand action.

the child when walking, either on deck or in the water, so assistance can be provided if needed.
- Never lift a child with muscular dystrophy by the arms or armpits. (No swimmer should ever be lifted by arms alone. Serious shoulder damage to the swimmer can result.)
- Do not lift a child alone - learn proper lifting techniques. Parents, and the child, can help with this.

Orthopedic Impairments

Orthopedic impairments are injuries or impairments of bones, joints, muscles, and tendons, which impede motor function. Some orthopedic impairments are temporary (a sprained ankle, for instance); some, such as an amputation, are permanent. The individual may have mobility problems, due to decreased muscular strength and endurance, impaired balance, paralysis, and/or lower physical fitness level. A person who is paralyzed may use a wheelchair for mobility on land.

Decreased strength, impaired balance, low fitness level.

Any person who has limited mobility on land has greater freedom of movement in the water. This increased freedom and independence are really enjoyable, and provide a great psychological boost. In addition, increased activity levels are possible, and aid in improving general fitness levels. Safety, fun, and swimming are obvious goals. Less obvious are functional goals - improved balance, range of motion, and physical fitness. Good activity programs can provide all of these.

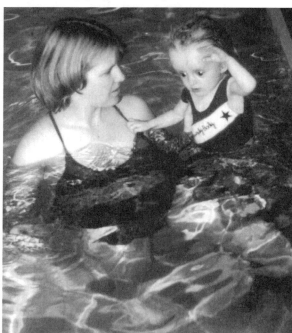

A child with osteogenesis imperfecta (brittle bones) finds water a great environment!   **Photos courtesy Fairfax County**

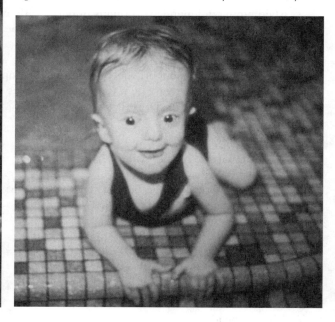

Balance, buoyancy, and propulsion

Effect on Aquatic Participation

When teaching children who have orthopedic impairments, primary areas needing adaptation are buoyancy, balance, and propulsion. For example, a child who has one leg amputated may be more buoyant (primary buoyancy is from the lungs, and legs tend to drag us down), but have less balance, since the body tends to roll away from the side of amputation. The individual may also have propulsion differences, since kicking with only one leg provides a different propulsive force and direction. Some children learn to compensate for this rapidly, and some need help in learning counter-balance, buoyancy compensation, and hand propulsion-direction.

Freedom of movement

Independent mobility, effected by any means, is important. For one who has limited mobility on land, water can provide great freedom.

Some children who have lower paralysis also have limited bowel and bladder control. They may need to wear some type of garment (cloth, not disposables) under their swim suits. Check with the parents regarding a child's bowel and bladder control.

A child with some paralysis may have low skin sensitivity of the affected body part, and probably poor circulation. It is most important to avoid injury (abrasions, scraping) to affected areas. A skin tear can be literally dangerous to a disabled person. If it becomes infected, it can be life-threatening. Any tear, even a minor one, could take months to heal; causing a skin-tear while putting a disabled swimmer in the water is simply not acceptable. Every surface that the swimmer comes in contact with must be smooth and free from any burrs. You must test every surface carefully. If there is any question about the texture of the surfaces, have your staff test them, doing slide-ins, before you use the areas for disabled persons. A reasonable accommodation is to use exercise pads covered with towels, or rubber mats of some type at pool side, for non-abrasive slide-in entries by persons with disabilities.

Never cause abrasions, scrapes or tears.

Orthopedic impairments can affect a child's balance, muscular strength, range of motion, and cardiovascular efficiency. Individuals who have paralyzed legs (paraplegia) often have good upper body strength, because of reliance on arms for much of their activity.

Weight bearing activities may be impossible on land for some individuals, but be possible in the water - water is 70 % more dense than air, and thus much more supportive. Check with the parent, to learn what activities (if any) should be avoided.

If a child can perform a swimming stroke in a correct and efficient manner, that should be encouraged. Efficient swimming techniques will always be advantageous, particularly if the individual wishes to become a competitive swimmer.

Teaching Suggestions

- Teach recoveries carefully (see section on muscular dystrophy).

- Bobbing and breathing activities (Adventure 1) are important, and help improve cardiovascular efficiency.

- Avoid allowing the child to become chilled or over-fatigued.

- If a child cannot walk unassisted on land, independent walking in the water will be an important, exciting achievement. Remind the child to scull or fin with the hands, to help provide balance. Allow some walking time each lesson - and smile; give some positive feedback!

- Underwater arm recovery may be easier than over-the-water recovery, because it affects balance and buoyancy less. Use flotation devices if necessary, to provide balance.

- Strokes on the back are sometimes easier, at first, since they minimize breathing problems, and retain visual references.

- If teaching a child with frail (brittle) bones (osteogenesis imperfecta), remember any impact is dangerous, even just jumping in from the deck.

- Individuals who have paralyzed legs may have sensitive feet, and may need to wear socks, scuba booties or pool shoes while swimming.

- Learn proper lifting and transferring techniques, both for your own sake and for the sake of the swimmer.

- Hand paddles or fins are sometimes used, to increase resistance and provide both propulsion and strength development. Make sure equipment fits properly, and does not create friction sores.

Pool shoes made for water exercise are great!

Never lift a swimmer by his or her arms alone.

Visual Impairments

A visual disability is an inability to carry out specific visual tasks. Visual abilities are called impaired if they measure below 20/40, or are impaired in depth perception, muscular action, or peripheral vision. A child who has a corrected vision of 20/200 or less is classified as legally blind. Most people with visual impairments are not totally blind, but can see light and dark, and discern movement.

Don't assume a child sees a demonstration- get feedback to verify understanding.

Functional abilities of children with visual impairments will vary greatly, depending upon amount of sight loss, experience in the environment, and training. Children who are totally blind may have mannerisms called blindisms — they may rock back and forth, rub their eyes, or wave their hands in front of their face. Blindisms usually disappear when an individual has learned mobility and achieved a degree of comfort in the environment — they are not inherently related to blindness. Activity and movement experiences are very important in developing this comfort in space.

Hearing and touching are important to the child's understanding - when one sense is gone or limited, input from the other senses becomes vital. This use of the other senses for information develops with experience and is not an automatic compensation.

Most blind children today have had mobility training, and are accustomed to being guided or assisted in specific ways. Usually it is not being led by the hand, but rather walking beside you, being guided by touching your elbow.

It is always advisable to warn a child with a visual impairment about hazards, direction changes, and steps - and be sure to say whether the steps go up or down!

It is highly likely your vocabulary will need to change. We usually speak to people as if they can see items to which we refer, and thus we are non-specific in our conversation. It doesn't do much good to warn a person who is blind by saying "Look out!" You must say what it is to look out for! If this comment doesn't make sense to you, try going blindfolded for a full day, and it will!

Practice specific language

One thing you don't need to change is your use of the words see and look. People with visual impairments use those words all the time, and they do see, and look - they simply do so with other senses and other actions than with their eyes.

Effect on Aquatic Participation

Use tactile and auditory cues

A visual impairment has little effect on a child's ability to swim and engage in aquatic activities. Sometimes, people who have visual impairments have trouble swimming in a straight line, because of the absence of visual cues. It is probable the main effect is upon the instructor - the need to give auditory and tactile cues, and to be specific in language.

Sometimes, children with visual impairments seem more sensitive to chlorine and other chemicals in the pool water. It is appropriate to allow the child to wear swim goggles, which not only protect the eyes but can increase visibility and enhance the underwater experience.

If your program is large, and thus perhaps very noisy, a child who is visually impaired may get confused by the sound bombardment. Usually, however, the child is good at masking out unwanted noise, and tunes in on the teacher's voice.

With even a mild visual impairment, a child may not be able to benefit from visual cues. Auditory and tactile cues must be used - simple explanations and coactive modeling are most effective. (Modeling refers to the act of moving the child's arm or leg in the desired pattern of motion, or of letting the child feel your arm as it does the desired motion.)

Hazards in the environment must be eliminated. Cluttered decks, half-open doors, newly placed benches and chairs are all hazardous to children with visual impairments.

Teaching suggestions

- Explain the environment to a child who has a severe visual impairment, not only to minimize hazards, but to improve comfort level. Walking around the pool, and letting the child experience the distance and configuration will help him/her measure the environment and learn where the deep end and dangers are found.

- Use auditory and tactile cues, and do modeling.

- If you can put some type of noise-maker (i.e., radio) at the shallow end of the pool, it helps children in locating and orienting to the environment.

- Don't offer too much help; it is always appropriate to ask a child if help is wanted. Some children prefer independence in all things, some appreciate a bit of help. Ask.

- Don't expect a child to benefit from demonstrations, even if the individual appears to see and understand. Ask the child to show you how the arms moved, and then do modeling if needed.

- Never leave a visually impaired child standing alone in unknown space, without some contact. A chair, a fence, the pool side, another person can provide the needed contact.

- It is appropriate for you to tell a child when you approach, and identify yourself. You will find that the child will quickly learn the sound of your voice, and will not need to be told who you are. You should also let a child know when you intend to touch.

- Even in a noisy aquatic environment, a child with a visual impairment can be adept at sound location, and swim toward the sound of your voice.

- Either hold the child's hands, or provide other tactile reference (the side of the pool, or a rope), the first few times he/she submerges - remember how important their hearing is to them; they lose it too, underwater!

- Remember the importance of specific praise and feedback.

Movement activities and opportunities for physical activity are very important for individuals with visual impairments. Such activities greatly increase the individual's comfort in space, and ability to function in the environment. Swimming can play an important part in this development.

There are many disabilities which affect the perceptual motor function of children, and it is the function, not the disability, which should be the focus of our attention as we teach swimming. In the past, entirely too much emphasis was placed upon impairment — upon handicaps and inability. Individuals who had an impairment were labeled "handicapped", and the label itself created certain "perceptual sets" in the minds of the population at large. Individuals were regarded as incompetent, unable to care for themselves, unable to learn, and almost every other negative concept one could imagine. The label created the handicap. When we hear a label, our brains conjure up a list of expected behaviors or characteristics (a perceptual set), and "attach" them to the person wearing the label. Of course, the majority of the characteristics on the list never apply to any one individual. Many things have happened to help change that perspective — legislation, the extreme competence of wheelchair athletes, increased visibility and the everyday achievement of persons with disabilities, and the emphasis in our society on the rights of individuals. Progress has been made, but more is needed. Inclusion of children with disabilities in the **Learn to Swim Program** is a positive step toward removing these prejudices, and promoting equal opportunity for all individuals in our society.

In all of your teaching, remember -

First, **a child**

Second, **a child who has varying abilities**

Third, **a child who has a disability**

AQUATIC GAMES

Water: Fun for Everyone!

Learning should be fun. All of us tend to repeat activities that are enjoyable, and not to repeat activities that are not enjoyable. Unfortunately, many people believe that "games are for children"— that when one becomes an adult, one must always behave in a serious fashion. We adults have too often forgotten how to play games. But water should be fun for everyone, and children learn through play and games. The Learn to Swim Program is built upon this philosophy — Swish and the Adventures are wonderful play. In addition to the Adventures, instructors may wish to incorporate other age-appropriate games into the water learning experience. Using the play and games approach, results for the students will include faster learning, increased motivation, and a capacity to enjoy aquatic activities for a lifetime; for the instructor, a renewed joy in play — a highly appropriate adult activity!

Purposes of Games in Aquatics

When used as a teaching tool, games can serve many purposes. In addition to those mentioned above, games can be used to do the following:

Motivation and lifetime aquatics!

- increase watermanship
- increase interest
- provide skill practice
- provide competition
- provide opportunities for success
- reduce apprehension
- create an atmosphere of fun

Reduce fear, increase water comfort

A single game may provide many of these benefits, or it may provide only a few. Often, the single purpose of a game is to reduce the apprehension or fear of the aquatic environment. This is especially true when teaching beginning students, and may be doubly important for students who have a disability. It is not at all unusual for a child to successfully attempt an activity in a game, which was not attempted in a "regular lesson" due to fear. In fact, the best learning situation for children is when games and play are used as the total teaching approach — they are the lesson.

Adapting Traditional Games

Some aquatic activities are fun while at the same time they enhance the participants social, emotional, and physical (psycho-motor) development. These activities can be enjoyed by non-disabled swimmers and swimmers who have disabilities, so they are especially useful in inclusive (mainstream) programs. The games can be adapted to the swimmer's abilities. Many traditional land-based games can be adapted to the aquatic environment. Modifications can be made for the specific needs of the children playing the game.

Leading Games

The key to success in using the game approach is the teacher's attitude — the game is only as good as its leader. If you are enthusiastic, and enjoy playing games, your students will enjoy them also. A good leader will give simple, concise instructions, and maintain a playful, enthusiastic attitude — make it your party, too!

Safety in Aquatic Games

It's your party too!

There are additional factors that affect children's safety as they play games. While it is true that children may forget their fears while playing games, they may forget other things, as well! Safety rules must apply during games also, and teachers and aides must be observant, and quick to help a child who looses his or her balance, or who becomes frightened at unexpected splashing or other activities. Games need to be chosen because they are appropriate to the age level and skill level of the children, both for enjoyment and safety purposes. Equipment must be maintained in good condition, and used in safe ways. Games must be conducted in water of safe depth, and lifeguards should be alerted to specifically guard against children walking, floating or swimming beyond a safe depth. During all activities, the teacher should stand between the children and deep water, and always facing the children.

The Play Approach and Games as a Teaching Method

The play approach of the Learn to Swim Program with Swish the Fish is especially well suited to reducing the child's fear of the water and new situations. Including other games can enhance this effect. The games which follow are particularly well suited to beginner swimmers. Some are developmental in nature, incorporating aspects of perceptual motor development; some are designed to reinforce specific aquatic skills. Some of the games require equipment, some do not. All games included here are for use with pre-beginner or beginner level students, in water chest deep or no more than shoulder deep for the children.

Each game has a title, a purpose, and a description. If a game is more suitable for children who have a specific disability, that information is included in the purpose. There are several books listed in the resource / reference section, page 155, which include many other aquatic games.

GAMES

Name of the game: Chin Ball

Prebeginners
and beginners

Purpose: Water adjustment. Useful primarily for children who can walk. Incorporates balance, kinesthetic awareness, spatial awareness.

Equipment: Tennis balls

Description: Children walk across the pool, each pushing a ball to another child with their chins. (No hands touching the balls). This can be used as a relay, once the children are sufficiently comfortable in the water.

Name of the game: Huff 'n Puff Race

Prebeginners
and beginners

Purpose: Water adjustment. Also useful in developing breath control. Like Chin Ball, it is useful primarily for children who can walk, and incorporates balance, kinesthetic awareness and spatial awareness.

Equipment: Ping pong balls

Description: Children walk across the pool, blowing the ball in front of them, not touching the ball with their hands. This also can be used as a relay race, when the children are comfortable in the water.

Name of the game: Sponge Play

Young
prebeginners

Purpose: Water adjustment
Equipment: Sponges (small or medium size) Plain rectangular sponges may be used, or the geometric shape sponges or nerf balls make a nice change.

Description: With the child one-on-one with an instructor, aide or parent, the following sequence is used:
1. Instructor submerges sponge, brings it up and squeezes out the water.
2. Instructor hands sponge to child, says "Now you do it".
3. Child submerges sponge, brings it above water and squeezes out water.
4. Instructor submerges sponge, brings it up and washes own face with it.
5. Child does same.
6. Instructor submerges sponge, hands it to child and says "Put it on my head and squeeze it out!". (and laughs when it happens!)
7. Instructor submerges sponge, hands it to child, and says "Put it on your head and squeeze it". (and rewards child appropriately when it happens!)

Name of the Game: Sponge Toss

Prebeginners
and beginners

Purpose : Water adjustment. Uses laterality skills, kinesthetic awareness, eye-hand coordination, visual and auditory response.

Equipment: Sponges. Do not use extra large sponges — they can become dangerously heavy when saturated.

Description: With participants in a circle, sponges are tossed back and forth in a game of catch. If done with children who are blind, participants should let the visually impaired children know when a sponge will be tossed to them. With older children, this game often deteriorates into a sponge fight, and then into a "get the teacher" game — none of which is a problem unless some children are very fearful, or the sponges are too large. Properly controlled, it is fun and does help with water adjustment.

Name of the game: Sink the bucket

Purpose: Water adjustment,

Equipment: Plastic bucket

Description: With children in a circle, the bucket floating in the middle, the children try to sink the bucket by splashing water into it. The teacher retrieves the bucket if and when it sinks or is full.

Name of the game: Simon Says

Purpose: Water adjustment, auditory discrimination, body awareness. Good for young children, and those with developmental delay or mental retardation.

Equipment: None

Description: With children in a circle or in random positions, the leader tells children to copy everything she or he does, if the command is preceded by "Simon Says". Those who forget, and do a motion not proceeded by "Simon Says", are pointed out and admonished "But Simon didn't say....". As a land based game, this has often been used as an elimination game, where children who make a mistake are eliminated from play. Since elimination games often disqualify those who most need the activity, they are best modified in such a way that the child who makes a mistake is not eliminated, but remains in the game.

Name of the game: Splash Ball

Purpose: Water adjustment. Uses balance and coordination.

Equipment: Oversize or regular size beach ball

Description: Children in a circle splash the ball without touching it, to move it away from themselves and toward the center of the circle.

Name of the game: Obstacle Course

Purpose: Water adjustment, reinforcement of movement concepts, kinesthetic and spatial awareness, directionality, visual discrimination.

Equipment: A post or a standard, hula hoops, ropes, Snapwalls, other play equipment.

Description: An obstacle course is set up in a segment of shallow water, with obstacles to step over, move around, go over and under, in and out, and through. Hula hoops, both floating and anchored to be vertical, are useful at several points of the course. Ropes are good for going under and over. A small child, or a non-ambulatory child, can be carried through the course. However, maximum benefit in terms of perceptual motor performance will be derived only if the child's movements are self-initiated.

Name of the game: Hokey Pokey

Purpose: Practice movement concepts, body awareness, laterality, balance. Group activity, fun. Water adjustment activity.

Equipment: None

Description: Group forms a circle, instructor sings the Hokey Pokey song and leads the group in the actions that go with the song: You put your right hand in,
> You put your right hand out,
> You put your right hand in, and you shake it all about,
> You do the Hokey Pokey and you turn yourself around,
> That's what it's all about!

It is usual to do right hand/left hand, right foot/left foot, head, backside, and whole self.

Name of the game: Magic Circle

Purpose: Water adjustment, laterality, directionality, spatial and body awareness, balance. Good for class control.

Equipment: Bunge cord, securely spliced and taped into a circle of 8 feet in diameter.

Description: Standing in shallow water, all children hold the rope with both hands. Teacher gives instructions, as "Lift the rope high", "Push the rope low", "Climb over the rope", "Hold the magic rope and walk around the circle", "Go in the magic circle", etc.

Prebeginners and beginners.

Name of the game: Who Can?

Purpose: Water adjustment, skill practice. Single component skills may be necessary for those children who have difficulty with sequencing.

Equipment: None

Description: Children in circle or random positions. Instructor calls out "Who can....
... splash with their hands
.... put their face in the water
.... blow bubbles
.... do a front float
etc. (Questions depend on skill level of swimmers.) Children respond by performing the skill/activity. Be careful to phrase the question as "Who can? ", not "Can you...?" The "Can you" question often leads to a "No!" response.

Prebeginners and beginners.

Name of the game: Pick the Flowers

Purpose: Encourage submersion, practice control of body position

Equipment: Plastic flowers, weighted with lead sinkers or by other means, are scattered around the pool bottom. The area may be roped off with buoyed lines.

Description: The activity may be done as a "Who can pick a flower" question, or may be done as a contest, seeing who can pick the most flowers. Since the flowers stand up from the bottom, they are easier to "pick" than items lying flat on the bottom. Thus, the activity can be done successfully by children having less skill in underwater swimming, and less balance and control of body position in the water.

Beginners
Journey 1
skills needed.

Name of the game: Marco Polo

Purpose: Practice balance, buoyancy, auditory response.

Equipment: None, or blindfolds.

Description: This is a tag game, in which "It" is blindfolded or has eyes closed. Children are in random positions around prescribed area. When "It" calls out "Marco", other children must respond with "Polo". Child who is It attempts to locate other children by sound, and tag them. Children may swim underwater or move from the position where they responded, but they must all respond. If a blind child is "It", then all children should be blindfolded.

Beginners or
Journey 2
skills desirable.

Name of the Game: Musical Hula Hoops

Purpose: Gross motor performance, auditory discrimination, kinesthetic awareness, fun

Equipment: Hula hoops

Description: Hoops are afloat randomly on the water. Leader sings or otherwise plays music. Like musical chairs, each child must find and get into a hoop when the music stops. Child who fails to get in a hoop is eliminated. As with other games, this can change to a non-elimination game, by allowing

Beginners or
Journey 2
participants.

more than one child in a hoop. A fun variation is to remove one hoop after each stop, until the hoops become too crowded. The game may be varied by ruling different ways to enter the hoop - feet first, head first, from underwater, etc.

Name of the game: Treasure hunt

Journey 2 & 3 participants.

Purpose: Practice underwater swimming, eye-hand coordination, balance, following directions, sequencing, spatial orientation, breath control.

Equipment: A variety of sinkable objects- toys, pennies, poker chips.

Description: A group game in which many sinkable objects are tossed into the pool. At the start signal, players sit or surface dive, collecting objects until the stop signal. Player with the most objects wins the hunt/relay.

All of these games, and many others, can be played in the water with young beginners, and are appropriate for classes which include children who have disabilities. Many playground games, such as Dodge Ball, Red Rover, Circle Tag and others, can be enjoyed in the water. The games included here should give you a start toward adapting and using additional games. The books listed on page 155 include many other games. Use your imagination and create your own games, and ask the children to describe or create games. Remember, children learn through play.

The qualities of children - the joy of discovery, the curiosity, the enthusiasm, the spontaneity - are qualities which we should foster, and which we should also try to retain in ourselves. We should not degrade these qualities as "immature", but rather value them and strive to retain them into our adulthood. Playing games can help us do so: thus play is very appropriate adult activity, also. So, play games!

If you are interested in learning more about teaching children and adults who have disabilities, the following publications can provide much additional information.

Adapted Aquatics - To laugh...   **to learn...**   **... to share.**

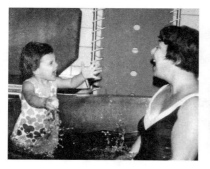 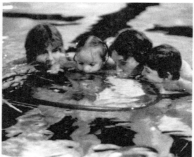 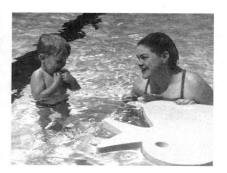

ADAPTED AQUATICS
RESOURCE MATERIALS

Canadian Red Cross Society. (1990) Adapted Aquatics: Promoting Aquatic Activities for All. Ottawa, Ontario. Canadian Red Cross Society

Cordellos, Harry.(1987) Aquatic Recreation for the Blind .Berkeley, CA. LaBuy Printing.

CNCA. Annotated Bibliography- Adapted Aquatics Cincinnati, OH.: Council for National Cooperation in Aquatics

CNCA National Aquatics Journal. Published quarterly, this journal contains many articles on the subject of adapted aquatics. Reprints and an index are available.

Fait,H.F. & Dunn, J.M. (1992). Special physical education: Adapted, individualized, and devel--opmental. Dubuque, IA.Wm.C. Brown.

Langendorfer, S. and Bruya, L., (1995) Aquatic Readiness. Champaign, IL, Human Kinetics

Miner, Maryalice. (1980) Water Fun. Englewood Cliffs, NJ. Prentice Hall

O'Rourke T.J.. A Basic Course in Manual Communication. Silver Spring, MD. National Association of the Deaf

Riekehof, Lottie. (1963) Talk to the Deaf. Springfield, MO. Gospel Publishing

Shank, Carolyn. (1983) A Child's Way to Water Play. Champaign,IL Leisure Press

Sherrill, Claudine.(1990). Adapted physical education and recreation: a multidisciplinary approach. Dubuque, IA . Wm.C. Brown.

Winnick, Joseph. (Ed) (1995) Adapted Physical Education and Sport. Champaign, IL. Human Kinetics.

YMCA of the USA (1986) Aquatics for Special Populations.
        Champaign, IL. Human Kinetics YMCA Program Store

For information on the Americans with Disabilities Act, you may contact the following:

U.S. Dept of Justice, Civil Rights Division
Office on the Americans with Disabilities Act
P.O.Box 66118
Washington, D.C. 20035-6118

Equal Employment Opportunity Commission
1801 L St. NW
Washington, DC 20507

Department of Transportation
400 Seventh St. SW
Washington, DC 20590

Federal Communications Commission
1919 M ST. NW
Washington, DC 20554

Architectural and Transportation
Barriers Compliance Board
1111 18th St. NW Suite 501
Washington, DC 20036

BOMA International
1201 New York Ave NW, Suite 300
Washington, DC 20005
(Publishes an ADA Compliance Guidebook)

ADAPTED AQUATICS GLOSSARY

Auditory — Having to do with the sense of hearing.

Balance — Ability to maintain equilibrium.

Bilateral — Having two sides: an awareness of sidedness.

Blindisms — Movements of the hands or body made by some blind persons.

Cardiovascular — Involving the heart and blood vessels.

Central Nervous System — The brain and the spinal cord.

Chromosome — The part of the cell that contains the genes.

Coactive — Moving together. Teacher and student moving arms together.

Cognitive — The mental process or faculty of knowing, of understanding.

Congenital — Present from birth: having been born with.

Contraction — Tightening / shortening of a muscle: reduction in size.

Contracture — Permanent contraction of a muscle.

Directionality — Knowledge of, or ability to move in, various directions.

Disability — An inability to do specific tasks, as a consequence of impairment.

Down Syndrome —A set of symptoms caused by a chromosome abnormality.

Finning — Moving the hands and forearms away from and then back toward the body, usually when in the supine position.

Flexibility — The ability to bend. Bending without breaking. Pliable.

Hemiplegia — Paralysis on one side of the body.

Hyperactive — Exceptionally active. Constant overactivity.

Hypertonicity — Excessive tone or tension of the muscles.

Impairment — Loss or abnormality of structure or function.

Information Processing — Ability to understand and correctly interpret sensory input.

Integrated skills — Highest level of laterality skills: arms,legs, and body can move in different patterns, planes, or rhythms at the same time.

Kinesthetic Awareness — Awareness of the body, body parts, and how they move.

Laterality — Sidedness. Knowledge of left and right.

Lipreading — Speech reading. Discerning words by watching lip movement.

Locomotor — Movement from one place to another.

Modeling — Moving student's arms/legs through desired pattern of motion.

Motoric — Movement. A part or system that causes movement.

Orthopedic — Having to do with bones, joints and muscles: locomotor structures.

Paralysis — Loss of function, sensation, or voluntary motion.

Paraplegia — Paralysis of lower portion of the body and the legs.

Perceptual Motor — The process of interpreting and responding to sensory input.

Perseverating — Inability to stop responding to a stimulus.

Physiological — Pertaining to the body, its parts and functions.

Prone — Lying face down. Floating face down in water.

Psychological — Having to do with the brain and behavior.

Quadriplegia — Paralysis of all four extremities and much of the body.

Rehabilitation — Process leading to fullest possible function.

Reinforcement — Anything that increases the likelihood of a behavior being repeated. A desired reward is positive reinforcement.

Respiration — The act of breathing.

Sculling — Moving the hands in a figure 8 motion.

GLOSSARY - CONTINUED

Self-image — A person's concept of, or ideas about, himself/herself.

Sequencing — Doing a number of things that follow one another

Spasticity — Convulsion of the muscles

Spatial awareness — Ability to perceive distance and location in space. Comprehension of one's position in space.

Startle response—A spastic muscle response to unexpected noise or actions

Structured environment— An environment in which expectations and activities are regular and predictable.

Supine— Positioned on the back

Tactile— Having to do with the sense of touch

Tonic neck thrust— A semi-fixed position in which the head is thrust back, the chin is raised.

Tonicity— Tension of the muscles

Visual discrimination— Ability to choose accurately (discern differences) between objects seen.

Appendix A
EARLY CHILDHOOD DEVELOPMENT

Changes in the child's motor movement from birth:

Infant (6-18 months)
- Primitive reflexes, gradually disappear about 6 months.
- Posture and equilibrium reactions gradually appear.
- Voluntary motor milestones
- Fine motor skills sequentially able to reach then grasp.

Toddler (18-36 months)
- Gross motor skills-begin with awkward basic skills, gradually become smooth with improved patten (walk, jump, bounce jump, gallop, run)
- Fine motor skills-grasp tools (feeding and scribbling)
- Fundamental motor skills-basic, awkward, and unskilled. Little control over force or accuracy (throw, strike, kick)

Preschooler (3-5 years)
- Locomotor skills-improved walking, running, hopping, jumping, sliding, galloping.
- Fundamental motor skills-become competent in throwing, striking, kicking. Begin catching, swinging and climbing.
- Fine motor skills-improved drawing and coloring, may begin writing letters, using scissors.

Changes in the child's thinking from birth to 6 years:

Infant
- Memory-shifts from immediate events to recent occurrences.
- Knowledge-links events together without action, begins to know that one event causes another.
- Object permanence-at about 6 months, existence of an object out of sight is understood; stranger/separation anxiety results.
- Language-sounds and babbles evolve into single-syllable words, learns own name, names of family members, objects.

Toddler
- Memory-expanded beyond infancy. Begins to remember past, dependent on oral memory.
- Knowledge-can think abstractly, very egocentric (self-centered) and thinks all things are alive.
- Language-may say more than 20 words by second birthday, often is hard to understand, likes repetition of stories, uses combinations of two words or more.

Preschooler
- Memory-has sense of past and future, but not like an adult. Remembers through speech, can recite songs and rhymes.
- Knowledge-intelligence develops, fears and worries are based on primitive thinking patterns.
- Language-vocabulary includes commonly used words and sentences, questions, can count, very pragmatic and literal, may not understand humor or sarcasm.

Changes in the child's feelings and perceptions.

Infant
- Feelings-general and without specific stimuli.
- Perceptions-linked directly to actions and stimuli.
- Expressions-cries, smiles and laughs.

Toddler
- Feelings-basic, but linked to increasing language skills; may use movement to communicate feelings.
- Perceptions-limited discrimination of stimuli; poor selective attention, unable to integrate different senses.

Preschooler
- Feelings-self-centered, but may be empathetic with others; expresses some feelings vocally.
- Perceptions-increasing discrimination of stimuli, limited attention to adult-specified tasks; begins to integrate senses.

EARLY CHILDHOOD DEVELOPMENT CONTINUED

Changes in the child's play and socialization

Infant
- Socialization-only smiles and vocalizes through first 6 months.
- Play-manipulates objects; independent explorations; singing may be soothing.

Toddler
- Socialization-linked with language development; self-centered.
- Play-independent, or with other children; difficult to share toys with others; simple drills may be enjoyable; structured games are beyond ability; enjoys songs and rhymes.

Preschooler
- Socialization-continues to develop, but incomplete; learns basic rules to interact with adults and peers.
- Play-major approach to learn and develop; small groups often use dramatic and expressive play; may use simple games.

Changes in the child's swimming behavior

Infant
- Breath control-reflexive breath holding; may develop ability to sequentially hold breath, then submerge.
- Leg actions-infrequent voluntary leg movements may develop into propulsive kicking actions (pedaling, running, frog-kick)
- Arm actions-arms held passively at side or overhead; may develop into splashing or weak paddling movements.
- Body position-body position in water is controlled by adult; may progress to body position controlled by child.

Toddler
- Breath control-active submersion; may blow bubbles; dislikes adult control of submersion.
- Leg actions-pedaling action may change to simple flutter kick or frog kick action.
- Arm actions-paddling movements may develop into alternating pulling actions, with most of the force downward.
- Body position-child prefers vertical position in water; often dislikes back position.

Preschooler
- Breath control-experienced preschooler can submerge for several seconds, swim underwater and open eyes to retrieve objects; most children still lift head straight up out of the water to get breath. Inexperienced preschooler shows fear and dislike for water in the face, but distractions can calm fear.
- Leg actions-effectiveness of kick depends on body position; individual preferences between flutter kick and breaststroke kick are often evident.
- Arm action- arm actions become more efficient; experienced child may progress to using overwater recovery for crawl stroke.
- Body position-head position determines body position; when head is raised, body becomes more vertical. Experienced child may submerge head and maintain a semi-horizontal position.

EARLY CHILDHOOD DEVELOPMENT CONTINUED

Developmental Skill Readiness Guidelines

Infant skills: (6-18 months)

	Objective of the skill:
Water adjustment	Readiness for entry; awareness of surroundings
Water entry	Safety
Front kick	Leg movement
Bubble blowing	Breath control, fun
Prone glide	Experience water support, independent movement
Underwater exploration	Underwater adjustment, breath control
Back float	Safety and relaxation
Arm movement	Stroke readiness
Combined skills	Coordinated movement
Rolling over	Safety, roll to back for air
Parent safety	Safety awareness, drowning prevention
Water exit	Safety

Toddler skills: (18-36 months) Objective of the skill:

Water adjustment	Readiness for entry; awareness of surroundings
Water entry	Safety
Front kick	Leg movement, independence, coordination
Bubble blowing	Breath control, fun
Prone glide	Experience water support, independent movement, forward movement, buoyancy, controlled glide/float
Underwater exploration	Underwater adjustment, breath control
Back float	Safety and relaxation
Back glide	Coordination, stroke readiness
Arm movement	Propulsion readiness
Combined skills	Coordinated movement
Rolling over	Safety, roll to back for air
Changing positions	Body control
Parent safety	Safety awareness, drowning prevention
Water exit	Safety

References:

The American Red Cross. 1988. American Red Cross Infant and Preschool Aquatic Program. The American National Red Cross, Washington, DC, 150 pp.

Langendorfer, S., Roberts, M., and Ropka, C. 1987. Aquatic Readiness: A Developmental Test. National Aquatics Journal 2 (3):8-12.

Appendix B
CPR PRACTICE CHECKLIST (NON-AQUATIC EMERGENCY)

Rescuer should perform bold type skills.
Partner/evaluator should prompt with italic commands, and look for correct performance.

PERFORMANCE/EVALUATION ⇓	PERFORMANCE TIPS ⇓

____**SURVEY THE SCENE**
    "The scene is safe"
____**CHECK FOR UNRESPONSIVENESS**
    "There is no response"
____**DIRECT SOMEONE TO CALL 911**

____**PUT ON GLOVES/UNIVERSAL PRECAUTIONS**

____**OPEN AIRWAY**...Rescuer should use head tilt-jaw thrust

____**CHECK FOR BREATHING** ....Rescuer should look at chest, ear near mouth
    "You do not see the chest rise or fall, or feel air coming out"
____**GIVE TWO SLOW, FULL BREATHS**........................Use ventilation mask (or BVM) with oxygen
    "The chest rose"
____**CHECK FOR PULSE FOR 5-10 SECONDS**...........At carotid artery(adult/child) brachial (infant)
    "You do feel a pulse"
____**START RESCUE BREATHING**............................1 Breath every 5 seconds(adult) 3:1 (child/infant)
    (after two cycles) "The air did not go in"
____**RE-TILT HEAD AND TRY BREATH AGAIN**...........Tilt forward, then re-open airway
    "The air still does not go in.
____**TURN HEAD TO THE SIDE**

____**5 HEIMLICH MANEUVERS**...............................Rescuer should line up with victim "knees to
                                            knees" for best thrust position
____**BLIND FINGER SWEEP**..............................(no blind sweep for child/infant, look only)
    (first cycle)"You do not find an object"
    (second cycle) "You remove an object"
____**RE-OPEN AIRWAY AND ATTEMPT TWO BREATHS**............ Use head-tilt/jaw thrust combination
    (first cycle) "The air still does not go in"
    (second cycle) " Air went in"
____**CHECK PULSE**
    "You cannot feel a pulse"
____**LOCATE HAND POSITION**..MINIMUM 2 fingers above xiphoid(adult),
                                            between nipple line (child/infant)
____**COMPRESSIONS** ....15 (adult) 5 (child/infant/2 rescuer)

____**VENTILATE**...2 breaths (adult) 1 breath (child/infant/2 rescuer)

____**COMPRESSIONS**

____**REPEAT CYCLE FOR ABOUT 1 MINUTE**
    "About a minute has gone by"
____**RECHECK PULSE AND BREATHING**......................... Check after compressions
    "There is still no pulse and no breathing
____**COMPRESSIONS**..Begin new cycle with compressions

____**VENTILATE**   **END PRACTICE SESSION**

Appendix C

CPR PRACTICE CHECKLIST (AQUATIC EMERGENCY)

Rescuer should perform bold type skills.

Partner/evaluator should prompt with italic commands, and look for correct performance

PERFORMANCE/EVALUATION ⇓	PERFORMANCE TIPS ⇓

____**EXTRICATE THE VICTIM**

____**CHECK FOR BREATHING**
  "There is no spontaneous breathing"
____**VERIFY THAT 911 HAS BEEN CALLED**

____**PUT ON GLOVES/UNIVERSAL PRECAUTIONS**

____**TURN VICTIM'S HEAD TO THE SIDE**

____**PERFORM 5 HEIMLICH MANEUVERS OR CONTINUE**......Line up knees to knees for best thrust
UNTIL WATER NO LONGER FLOWS FROM THE MOUTH

____**OPEN AIRWAY**...Rescuer should use head tilt-jaw thrust

____**GIVE TWO SLOW, FULL BREATHS**..Use ventilation mask (or BVM) with oxygen
  "The chest rose"
____**CHECK FOR PULSE FOR 5-10 SECONDS**.........................At carotid artery(adult/child) brachial (infant)
  "You do feel a pulse"
____**START RESCUE BREATHING**...1 Breath every 5 seconds(adult) 1:3 (child/infant)
  (after two cycles) "The air did not go in"
____**RE-TILT HEAD AND TRY BREATH AGAIN**...........................Tilt forward, then re-open airway
  "The air still does not go in."
____**TURN HEAD TO THE SIDE**

____**5 HEIMLICH MANEUVERS**...Rescuer should line up with victim
                                                                    "knees to knees" for best thrust
____**BLIND FINGER SWEEP**...(no blind sweep for child/infant, look only)
  (first cycle)"You do not find an object"
  (second cycle) "You remove an object"

____**RE-OPEN AIRWAY AND ATTEMPT TWO BREATHS**.............Use head-tilt/jaw thrust combination
  (first cycle) "The air still does not go in"
  (second cycle) " Air went in"
____**CHECK PULSE**
  "You cannot feel a pulse"
____**LOCATE HAND POSITION**..MINIMUM 2 fingers above xiphoid(adult),
                                                                    between nipple line (child/infant)
____**COMPRESSIONS** ....15 (adult) 5 (child/infant/2 rescuer)

____**VENTILATE**...2 breaths (adult) 1 breath (child/infant/2 rescuer)

____**COMPRESSIONS**

____**REPEAT CYCLE FOR ABOUT 1 MINUTE**
  "About a minute has gone by"
____**RECHECK PULSE AND BREATHING**...................................Check after compressions
  "There is still no pulse and no breathing
____**COMPRESSIONS**..Begin new cycle with compressions

____**VENTILATE   END PRACTICE SESSION**   162

Appendix D
CNCA GUIDELINES

AQUATICS ACTIVITY PROGRAMS FOR CHILDREN UNDER THE AGE OF THREE
(Council for National Cooperation in Aquatics)

1 AQUATIC PROGRAMS FOR CHILDREN UNDER THE AGE OF THREE YEARS, MOST APPROPRIATELY, SHOULD BE PROMOTED, DESCRIBED AND CONDUCTED AS WATER "ADJUSTMENT", "ORIENTATION", OR "FAMILIARIZATION" PROGRAMS. EMPHASIS SHOULD BE PLACED UPON THE NEED FOR YOUNG CHILDREN TO EXPLORE THE AQUATIC ENVIRONMENT IN ENJOYABLE, NON-STRESSFUL SITUATIONS THAT PROVIDE A WIDE VARIETY OF GAMES AND EXPERIENCES.

RATIONALE: Other terms, such as "drown proofing", "waterproofing" and "watersafe", often can suggest to parents and the general public that children can be safe in and around the water without careful supervision. In addition, the developmental literature supports the primary role of play activities and movement exploration in the acquisition of movement competence by young children.

2. WATER EXPERIENCE/ORIENTATION PROGRAMS SHOULD HAVE THE IN-WATER PARTICIPATION OF A PARENT, GUARDIAN, OR OTHER PERSON WHO IS RESPONSIBLE FOR AND TRUSTED BY THE CHILD.

RATIONALE: The parent is the first and primary teacher of the young child. As such, the parent must assume actual responsibility for the supervision and learning of the child. Aquatic programs, when properly structured, can provide an excellent type of parent-child learning environment. Programs conducted without parents in the water should be limited in size, and make every consideration for the safety and psychological comfort of the child.

3. THE PARTICIPATING PARENT, GUARDIAN OR OTHER RESPONSIBLE ADULT ASSUMES PRIMARY RESPONSIBILITY FOR MONITORING THE CHILD'S HEALTH BEFORE, DURING AND AFTER PARTICIPATION IN AQUATIC PROGRAMS. ALL CHILDREN, ESPECIALLY THOSE WITH KNOWN MEDICAL PROBLEMS, SHOULD RECEIVE CLEARANCE FROM THEIR PHYSI-CIAN PRIOR TO PARTICIPATION IN THE AQUATIC PROGRAM.

RATIONALE: The child's parent and physician are the persons who can best judge the child's medical and developmental readiness for exposure to a public swimming pool at an early age. There is disagreement among professionals about the benefits and detriments of the child's early exposure to the aquatic environment. The potential benefits of enhanced movement, socialization and parent-child interaction must be weighed against problems such as possible increased susceptibility to eye, ear respiratory and bacterial infections. More definitive research evidence is needed to assist parents and physicians in evaluating the child's readiness.

4. PERSONNEL DIRECTING AND OPERATING AQUATIC PROGRAMS FOR CHILDREN UNDER THREE YEARS OF AGE SHOULD HAVE TRAINING IN CHILD DEVELOPMENT AND PARENTING AS WELL AS AQUATICS, OR HAVE CONSULTANTS WHO HAVE BEEN TRAINED IN THESE AREAS. FULLY TRAINED AND QUALIFIED LIFEGUARDS MUST BE ON DUTY AT ALL TIMES DURING PROGRAMS.

RATIONALE: Because of the developmental differences in cognitive, psychomotor and affective domains between the young child and older children, the directors and teachers of these programs must have a well-founded understanding of child development. Because the programs usually involve both the parents and the children, a further understanding of parenting principles is also necessary. Finally, in spite of the presence of parents in the pool, it must be recognized that the instructor cannot assume lifeguarding responsibilities while teaching. A certified lifeguard in addition to the instructor is needed.

5. PARTICIPATION IN AQUATIC PROGRAMS BY NEONATES AND BY YOUNG CHILDREN LACKING PRONE HEAD CONTROL SHOULD BE LIMITED.

RATIONALE: While there is general disagreement among professionals and practitioners regarding the youngest age at which children should begin water experiences, there is some evidence suggesting that until the child can voluntarily control the head by lifting it 90 degrees when prone, they probably will gain little from the water experience, and may be more at risk of accidently submerging or swallowing water. Certain aquatic skills can successfully be introduced when the child demonstrates rolling over, crawling and creeping. Due to individual differences among young children, behavioral, rather than strict age, criteria are usually the most valid way to evaluate children for program participation.

6. CERTAIN TEACHING TECHNIQUES, SUCH AS DROPPING A CHILD FROM A HEIGHT, SHOULD BE STRICTLY PROHIBITED. OTHER PROCEDURES, SUCH AS FACE SUBMERSIONS, ESPECIALLY THOSE THAT ARE CONTROLLED BY AN ADULT, MUST BE LIMITED BOTH IN DURATION AND IN NUMBER FOR THE YOUNG CHILD.

RATIONALE: Dropping a child from any height is unnecessary and serves no reasonable purpose. In fact, it is extremely dangerous, as it may produce head,neck or organ damage to a young child, as well as introduce water and bacteria into the nose, ears and sinuses. There is also potential for psychological trauma in such an activity.

A growing number of recent clinical reports have implicated the practice of repeated submersions during aquatic programs in producing hyponatremia, or "water intoxification" in young children. Hyponatremia is a condition in which an electrolyte (especially sodium) imbalance results from the loss of electrolytes or rapid ingestion of fluids or both. The symptoms include such "soft" signs as irritability, crying and fussing, as well as more serious signs of vomiting,convulsions and coma. Despite claims that a young child has a "breath holding" or epiglottal reflex, both children and adults can swallow significant amounts of water while learning to swim. Due to the small body size and large skin area to body weight ratio of most children under 18 months of age, water ingestion can produce symptoms of hyponatremia, some of which may be going unnoticed by parents and teachers. Therefore, submersions by young children must be brief (one to five seconds), and few in number (less than six per lesson) while the child is initially learning. Once the child can initiate the submersions, AND can demonstrate competent breath control, submersions can become longer and more frequent. However, the parents and teachers still must be alert to bloated stomachs and "soft" signs that may indicate excessive water ingestion and incipient problems.
The condition of hyponatremia must be the focus of a concerted research effort to discover the extent and scope of its presence in infant swimming classes. Clinical and empirical evidence should be the basis for subsequent amendments to this guideline.

7. MAXIMUM IN-WATER CLASS TIME FOR INFANTS AND VERY YOUNG CHILDREN MUST NOT EXCEED THIRTY MINUTES.

RATIONALE: Most children benefit from shorter, but more frequent learning experiences. Limiting in-water time to less than 30 minutes should maximize the learning and enjoyment of children while avoiding fatigue, hypothermia, and possibly hyponatremia. One of the constant factors discovered in each clinical hyponatremia case was that children had been in the water far in excess of thirty minutes. Apparently, fatigue, chilling and excessive submersions all may contribute to hyponatremia.

8. WATER AND AIR TEMPERATURE MUST BE MAINTAINED AT SUFFICIENT LEVELS AND IN PROPER PROPORTION TO ONE ANOTHER TO GUARANTEE THE COMFORT OF YOUNG CHILDREN.

RATIONALE: Young children can become chilled more easily than adults and may have immature thermal regulatory systems. They also cannot enjoy the experience or learn optimally if chilled. There is no general agreement as to the proper level of water temperature in indoor pools. However, experience suggests that water temperature should be a MINIMUM of 82 degrees fahrenheit (86 is preferable) and that air temperature should be at least three degrees higher than the water temperature. Locker and changing room temperatures also should be maintained at warm levels. Failure to achieve these minimum standards should be a strong factor in cancelling or shortening classes.

9. ALL LAWS AND REGULATIONS PERTAINING TO WATER PURITY, POOL CARE, AND SANITATION MUST BE CAREFULLY FOLLOWED.

RATIONALE: Young children are extremely susceptible to disease. Utmost care in maintaining facilities in accord with bathing codes and water purity standards can prevent unnecessary outbreaks of disease and infections. Locker rooms and pool decks must be clean and free of clutter. Slippery surfaces and impeded walkways can be very dangerous to beginning and inexperienced walkers. Proper facilities for the changing and disposal of diapers and soiled clothing must be provided.

10. APPROPRIATE, BUT NOT EXCESSIVE CLOTHING SHOULD BE WORN BY YOUNG CHILDREN TO MINIMIZE THE SPREAD OF BODY WASTES INTO THE WATER.

RATIONALE: Fecal matter is aesthetically unattractive and potentially hazardous to other swimmers. Children should wear some type of tight-fitting but light weight apparel, perhaps covered by rubber pants. Heavier diapers can be both a health and safety hazard and should not be worn. Parents and instructors should monitor young children and remove them from the water if a bowel movement is apparent.

Council for National Cooperation in Aquatics
P.O.Box 68052
Cincinnati, OH 45206

Appendix E

The Exploration Program Participation Certificate Master art is located on the next page. Duplicate it as needed for the participants.

National Safety Council

National Recreation and Park Association™

ELLIS & ASSOCIATES

&

has completed the
National Safety Council
Jeff Ellis & Associates
Exploration Swim Program
on

Instructor

Facility

Facility Coordinator

Appendix F

The Challenge Participation Certificate Master art is located on the next page. Duplicate it as needed for the participants.

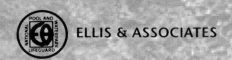 ELLIS & ASSOCIATES  National Recreation and Park Association

TM

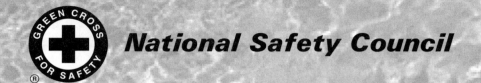 *National Safety Council*

_____

has completed the
National Safety Council
Jeff Ellis & Associates
Challenge Swim Program
on

_____

_____
Facility

_____
Facility Coordinator

_____
Instructor

Appendix G

The Adapted Participation Certificate Master art is located on the next page. Duplicate it as needed for the participants.

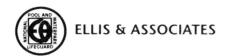 ELLIS & ASSOCIATES

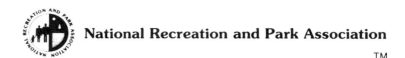 National Recreation and Park Association

TM

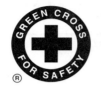 *National Safety Council*

_____

has completed the National Safety Council Jeff Ellis & Associates Adapted Swim Program on

_____

_____
Facility

_____   _____
Facility Coordinator   Instructor

Appendix H

The Fitness Challenge - Swim the Seven Seas Participation Certificate Master art is located on the next page. Duplicate it as needed for the participants.

INSTRUCTOR NOTES

INSTRUCTOR NOTES